Quick Workout for Beginners at Ease:

Simple Steps to Kickstart Your Fitness Journey – Your Easy Path to a Healthier You!

BY

Manuel N. Rank

Quick Workout for Beginners at Ease

Copyright:

Disclaimer:

The information provided in "Quick Workout for Beginners at Ease" is for general informational purposes only. While every effort has been made to ensure the accuracy and completeness of the content, the author and publisher make no representations or warranties of any kind, express or implied, about the suitability, reliability, or availability concerning the exercises, routines, or advice contained within this book. Always consult with a qualified healthcare professional before beginning any new exercise or dietary program. The author and publisher expressly disclaim any and all liability that may arise directly or indirectly from the use of this book. Your health and safety are paramount; use this information responsibly and in accordance with your individual circumstances

Quick Workout for Beginners at Ease

About the Author

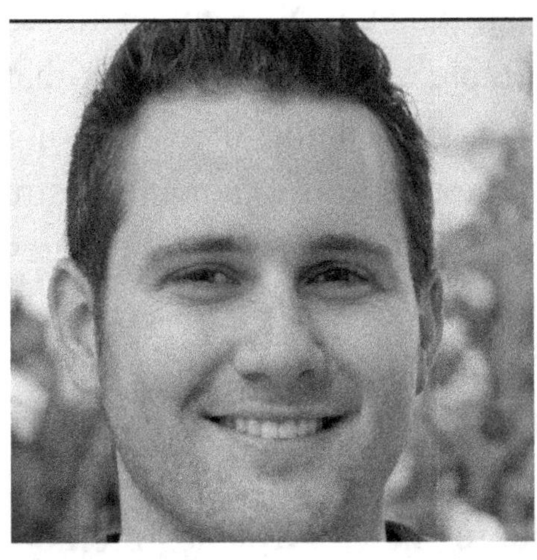

Meet Manuel N. Rank, the passionate creator behind "Quick Workout for Beginners at Ease." With a deep love for fitness and a commitment to making exercise accessible to everyone, Manuel N. Rank has crafted this guide as a friendly companion on your journey to a healthier lifestyle.

A certified fitness enthusiast and advocate for balanced well-being, Manuel N. Rank believes in the power of simple, effective workouts that seamlessly integrate into daily life. Drawing from personal experiences and a genuine desire to inspire others, Manuel N. Rank shares practical tips, motivational insights, and a holistic approach to fitness.

Beyond the pages of this book, Manuel N. Rank continues to explore new ways to promote health, positivity, and the joy of movement. Whether you're a fitness novice or someone seeking a fresh perspective on well-being,

Manuel N. Rank's goal is to empower you on your path to a more vibrant and active life.

Your adventure towards a healthier you is just beginning, and Manuel N. Rank is here to cheer you on every step of the way.

Quick Workout for Beginners at Ease

TABLE OF CONTENTS

Quick Workout for Beginners at Ease

INTRODUCTION

Welcome to the "Quick Workout for Beginners at Ease: Your Easy Path to a Healthier You!" This book is your go-to resource for starting a fitness journey that's not only easy and fun but also highly successful. Whether you're a complete newcomer to exercise or someone looking to refresh their routine, this book is designed to make fitness accessible for everyone.

In the pages that follow, you'll discover straightforward workouts tailored for beginners, focusing on aerobic fitness, strength training, core exercises, and more. No complicated routines or intimidating gym equipment – just easy-to-follow steps to kickstart your health and well-being.

Let's make fitness a part of your lifestyle without the hassle. Get ready to feel energized, confident, and at ease with your quick and achievable workout plan

Introduction to the importance of regular exercise

Ever stop to think about the magic regular exercise can bring to your life? "Quick

Workout for Beginners at Ease" is all about diving into that magic.

Picture this: more energy, a mood lift, and a healthier you—all from these easy, beginner-friendly workouts. It's not just about looking good (though that's a bonus); it's about feeling fantastic inside and out.

Life gets crazy, we get it. But taking a few moments for yourself with these quick exercises isn't just a checkbox on your to-do list; it's like giving yourself a daily gift of wellness. Let's make exercise a simple, joyful part of your routine, and discover the awesome changes it can bring. Ready to kickstart a healthier, happier you? "Quick Workout for Beginners at Ease" is your guide – let's do this!

Motivational tips for beginners

Beginning a fitness journey may be thrilling as well as difficult. In the section on motivational tips for beginners in "Quick Workout for Beginners at Ease," we explore ways to keep that initial enthusiasm burning bright. First off, let's banish the idea of perfection. Every step you take toward a healthier lifestyle is a win, no matter how small. Embrace progress, not perfection. It's about the journey, not just the destination.

Setting achievable goals is key. Think baby steps, not giant leaps. These small victories add up and keep you motivated. Plus, they're way less intimidating.

Surround yourself with positive vibes. Whether it's a workout buddy, a supportive friend, or even a playlist that gets you moving, having a positive environment can make all the difference.

And remember, it's okay to mix things up. If one workout doesn't click, try another. Finding what you enjoy makes staying active a whole lot easier.

Lastly, celebrate your wins. Did you finish a workout? High five! Small achievements deserve a moment in the spotlight.
Ready to keep that motivation high? "Quick Workout for Beginners at Ease" is your friendly guide to making fitness a lasting and enjoyable part of your life. Let's keep that motivation rolling!

19

Chapter 1

Warm-up wisdom

No one who cares about a car would take it straight from park to fifth gear or slam on the brakes while speeding down the highway at 60 mph. Even the best machine couldn't take that kind of treatment. Yet when exercisers are rushed, the first thing they'll skip is the warm-up or cool-down.

"People tend not to realize how important it is to slowly shift their gears into exercise and back out again," says Lance

Fujiwara, director of sports medicine at the Virginia Military Institute in Lexington. "Elite athletes, especially track athletes, may spend half an hour warming up and cooling down for every hour that they train." But novice athletes often neglect this crucial aspect of a workout, he says, "until they get injured."

Warming up reduces the risk of injury by preparing the body gradually for the stress of exercise. It boosts heart rate gradually, blood circulation quickly, breathing rate, and lung airway opening. By doing this, cardiac arrhythmias that can result from abruptly hard activity may be avoided. Additionally, muscles may process oxygen more quickly when body temperature rises. Additionally, bringing the temperature of the lubricating fluids, muscles, and tendons up gradually makes the body less prone to strain and more supple.

Physiologist Everett Harman holds out window putty to demonstrate the idea. "Cold putty will break, but once you warm it in your hands and soften it by kneading, it's pliable and elastic," says Harman, of the U.S. Natick, Massachusetts's Army Research Institute of Environmental Medicine. Similarly, a muscle that has been warmed by increased blood flow and body temperature is more pliable and less prone to injury. You'll feel less exhausted because warm muscles also store less lactic acid, a waste product of vigorous exercise.

But warming up is important for reasons other than its health benefits.

"Taking five or 10 minutes to ease into exercise gives you a chance to think about the training session ahead," says Steve Fleck, a sports physiologist at the U.S. Olympic Training Center in Colorado Springs. He states that if you dive straight into an activity without making this crucial mental shift, "your head might still be back in the office, and you might wind up doing something "foolish and getting hurt."

The most common warm-up mistake, Fleck says, "is that people stretch and think it's a warm-up. But it's not." In fact, he says, stretching should only be done after muscles are warm. To warm up properly, experts advise: * Do your activity at an easy pace for five to 10 minutes. Bikers can pedal slowly, runners can jog lightly, walkers can stroll, etc. (Warm up indoors if you're planning to go out into the cold, but get outside before you break a sweat.) * Warm up specific muscles you plan to use in your activity, (such as the shoulder for racquetball players or knees for basketball players) by using those muscles gently at first, then gradually increasing the intensity. * Once you're warmed up, lightly stretch major muscle groups and any muscles that are stiff or previously injured. The longer stretch should be saved for the end of your workout.

Also, remember to cool down after vigorous activity. Runners "like to kick out the last half-mile, then hit the showers," says Fleck. "But that's a bad habit." Intense exercise can cause the heart and lungs to work twice as hard, and if you stop moving suddenly, blood may pool in the dilated vessels of your legs. This strains the heart, causing dizziness and increasing your risk of abnormal heart rhythm.

Instead, slow down your pace gradually with five to ten minutes of light activity similar to your warm-up. If your activity has been strenuous, try walking with your hands behind your head to straighten your torso and encourage normal breathing. If you're too exhausted to walk, lie down on the ground and pump your legs. However, if you're this tired, you've probably worked out too hard.

• **Understanding the significance of warm-ups.**

Do you want to begin an exercise programme to get in shape and live a healthier lifestyle? An exercise routine may appear to be time consuming — but no matter what type of workout you choose or how hectic your schedule is, it is critical that you do not skip it warming up before your workout, or cooling down afterwards.

You'd be surprised how many people decide they don't need to warm up before working their core, or that skipping their cool-down after treadmill jogging is fine. Most of the time, it's not because people dislike doing the warm-up or cool-down, but rather because they want to save time. After all, the main part of the workout is what counts, right?

Unfortunately, it is not only the main part of your workout that is important — and people who skip the processes before and after a workout may be doing more harm than good to their bodies than they realize.

Why Is It Necessary to Warm Up and Cool Down?

A warm-up and a cool-down both involve performing exercises at a lower intensity and at a slower pace, which improves athletic performance, prevents injuries, and aids in exercise recovery.

Light jogging or cycling slowly on a bike are examples of warm-up activities. Warming up before exercise gets your cardiovascular system ready for physical activity by increasing blood flow to your muscles and raising your body temperature. It also helps to reduce the risk of injury because when your muscles are adequately warmed up, the movements, stretches, and strain you put on them during your workout are less likely to injure them. This also minimizes muscle soreness.

Cooling down after a workout is intended to gradually return your heart rate and blood pressure to their pre-exercise levels. Your heart rate has been much higher than normal during your workout, and it's important to ease it back down rather than abruptly stopping all motion. Cooling down also helps to regulate blood flow, which is especially important for endurance athletes like long distance runners. To safely cool down, gradually slow down your pace during the last 10 minutes of your workout — for example, if you're jogging, slow down to a brisk walk for the last 10 minutes.

Benefits of Warming Up
•Improved Performance
Warming up improves your performance in the following ways:
Warming up for 10 minutes with an easygoing activity increases blood flow to

your skeletal muscles and opens blood capillaries. Because your blood carries the oxygen your muscles require to function, increasing your blood flow is one of the best things you can do to prepare your muscles for a workout.

•Improved Oxygen Efficiency — When you warm up, oxygen is released from your bloodstream more readily and at higher temperatures. Because your muscles require more oxygen while exercising, it is critical to increase the availability of this oxygen through a warm-up activity.

•Faster Muscle Contraction/Relaxation — Warming up with physical activity raises your body temperature, which in turn, improves your nerve transmission and muscle metabolism. The end result? Your muscles will perform more quickly and efficiently.

•Injury Prevention

Warming up helps to prevent injuries by loosening your joints and increasing blood flow to your muscles, making them less likely to rip, tear, or twist in an unfavourable way during your workout. Stretching also helps your muscles prepare for the physical activities you're about to engage in.

•Mental Preparation

Warming up has the added benefit of focusing your mind on your body and physical activity as you go through the process. This focus will carry over into your training session to help you to improve your technique, coordination, and skill.

Benefits of Cooling Down

•Recovery

Lactic acid builds up in your system after intense exercise, and it takes time for your body to clear it out. Cooling down exercises (such as stretches) can help with this process of releasing and removing lactic acid, which can help your body recover faster after a workout.

•Reducing DOMS (Delayed Onset Muscle Soreness)

While some muscle soreness is to be expected after exercise, a significant amount of DOMS is extremely unpleasant and may prevent you from exercising in the future. A California State University study discovered that moderate intensity cycling after strength exercise helped to reduce DOMS. Cooling down after exercise helps to alleviate excessive muscle soreness, keeping you more comfortable and allowing your body to bounce back before your next work.

What Happens If You Don't Properly Warm Up and Cool Down?

Increased Risk Of Injury

Over 30% of injuries seen by sports medicine clinics are skeletal muscle injuries — which can be easily prevented by warming up and stretching.

Blood Pooling

If you abruptly stop exercising without cooling down, your muscles will stop contracting vigorously. This can cause blood to pool in your lower extremities, resulting in less pressure being pumped back to your heart and brain. As a result, you may feel dizzy, lightheaded, or faint.

Increased Stress On Cardiovascular System

Warming up allows you to gradually increase your heart rate and breathing rate to meet the demands of your workout. If you begin strenuous exercise without first warming up, you will put unnecessary strain on your heart and lungs.

A study of 44 men was conducted to investigate the effects of high intensity exercise on the heart. Without a warm-up, the subjects had to perform 10 to 15 seconds of intense exercise on a treadmill. The results showed that 70% of subjects had abnormal ECG readings because of the inadequate oxygen supplied to the heart — in essence, their hearts were not prepared to work at the high rates required for the strenuous exercises.

When you feel like you can't spare the extra 10 minutes to cool down after running, consider the impact it will have on your body. Those 10 minutes seem well spent when you consider that you're helping to prevent injuries, improve your performance, and aid in post-workout recovery.

•Easy warm-up exercises to prepare the body for workouts

Warming up your body before a workout can help you avoid injuries and maximise your workout time.

However, much of what we've been taught about warming up contradicts what our bodies actually require before a workout. It is critical to ensure stability throughout your movement during a proper warm-up to avoid injuries. There are several extremely beneficial movements you can perform to properly prepare your body.

Traditional stretching exercises that require you to push the limits of your range of motion, such as reaching for your toes, may be ineffective if not combined with other movements. These static stretches instruct your body to relax the muscles that protect your joints. This message isn't always helpful, especially when you need stabilising mechanisms during heavy lifting sessions.

Many people think of a warm-up as a way to get the blood flowing while making the muscles and tendons more pliable. While this is true to some extent, a warm-up should also activate your central nervous system (CNS), preparing it for the work ahead. One effective method is to perform dynamic movements similar to those you will perform during your workout. So, when deciding which movements to do during your warm-up, choose those that are most similar to what you will be doing during your training session. Bodyweight squats, for example, are an excellent warm-up movement for barbell squats, whereas banded rows help you connect to your back muscles before pulling exercises like barbell rows.

These more active movements will prime your CNS for the workout while also increasing your range of motion and stability. Keep in mind that each person's body and needs differ in terms of range of motion, joint stability, and mobility. When performing warm-up exercises, pay attention to your body; nothing should be painful. Aim for 3 to 4 warm-up movements, or more if you prefer. This should take you 5 to 10 minutes.

Warm-Up Exercises

Try these 10 warm-up exercises before your next workout.

- Bodyweight squats
- 90-90
- Bird dog
- Banded row
- Inchworms
- Wall angels
- Lunge with hip opener
- Gate opener
- Arm circles with reach
- Prone cobr

1. Bodyweight Squats

Bodyweight squats warm up the glutes and hip flexor muscles, as well as the quadriceps, abs, calves, and hamstrings. Bodyweight squats are an excellent warm-up if you intend to do any loaded squats during your workout. Squats, as a compound full-body movement, help to warm up multiple muscles at once and prepare your central nervous system for work.

Step-by-Step Instructions
•Position your feet hip-width apart, toes pointing straight ahead or slightly outward.
•Place your hands on your hips or in front of your body.

•Hinge your hips back, bend your knees, and keep your weight on your heels. Lower your hips toward the floor.
•Maintain a straight back.
Lower yourself until you feel a stretch in your quadriceps. Pause for one count before pushing through your heels and extending your hips back to the starting position.
•Repeat 10 times.

2. 90-90

Through internal and external rotation, the 90-90 movement will help open up the hips. While this may appear to be a passive stretch, it is actually an active stretch of the gluteus muscles.

If you feel any pinching pain in this position, stop immediately and consult a professional.

Step- by- step instructions

•Sit on the ground with your right leg 90 degrees in front of you and your left leg 90 degrees behind you.

•You should be able to sit up straight and tall.

•If you raise your left arm straight, your left knee and arm should line up, as should your hip and shoulder.

• To support your posture, place your right hand beside you, palm down, fingers pointing behind you.

•Pay close attention to your right (front) leg's knee and ankle. Stay if this is difficult as it is.

•Keep your chest up and lean forward to hover over your right knee. Instead of letting your knee rise off the ground, actively push the knee and ankle into the ground.

•You should feel a deep stretch. Hold for 5 seconds while actively pushing your knee and ankle into the ground. Return to an upright position.

•Repeat the movement five times before switching legs and doing it again on the opposite side.

3. Bird Dog

The bird dog exercise is great for getting your abs and lower back in shape. In preparation for your workout, this movement will activate the core muscles that support your spine. This exercise will also strengthen your glutes and hip flexors.

Step-by-Step Instructions

•Get down on all fours on the ground, knees under hips, wrists under shoulders.

•Contract your abs and maintain a neutral spine by drawing your shoulder blades back and down towards your hips.

•Raise and lengthen your left leg until it is straight back and parallel to the floor, while raising and straightening your right arm until it is parallel to the floor. Your head and shoulders should be straight and aligned.

•Return your arm and leg to the starting position slowly and switch sides.

•Repeat 10 times on each side.

4. Banded Row

Movements at the back of your body can be difficult to feel correctly. The mind-muscle connection is critical for proper form and results. A banded row will help you activate your back muscles. Warming up your shoulder joints and shoulder blades is another benefit of banded rows.

Step-by-Step Instructions

•Place a resistance band under your feet and grasp the handles. Your feet should be shoulder-width apart, with your toes slightly pointed out.

•Keep your knees slightly bent and your hips forward. Maintain a flat back and an engaged core.

•Pull the resistance band handles back, starting with your elbows and bringing your shoulder blades closer together. Hold the contraction in your upper back for one count.

•Return to the starting position slowly.

•Repeat 10 times more.

5. Inchworms

The inchworm exercise strengthens your front body muscles while stretching your back body muscles. This movement will engage your entire body, making it ideal for an active warm-up. Stabilising muscles in your shoulders, hips, glutes, quadriceps, and core will begin to fire up, preparing your body for your workout.

 Step-by-Step Instructions

•Take a natural stance and stand tall.

•Hinge from your hips and, if possible, touch the floor with your fingertips or palms.

•Walk your hands as far forward as you can without letting your hips sag while keeping your legs straight.

•Aim to finish in a plank position with your hands under your shoulders.

•Return your hands to your feet slowly and straighten to the starting position.
•Repeat 10 times more.

6. Wall Angel

Wall angels are an excellent dynamic stretching exercise for your spine, upper back muscles, and joints. This warm-up stretching movement can also help relieve achy and tight neck muscles. Wall angels put your thoracic spine and shoulder mobility to the test. If your workout includes squats, overhead pressing, or other exercises that require thoracic spine mobility, this movement is ideal.

Step-by-Step Instructions

•Stand against a wall, feet shoulder-width apart, and take two or three steps out. Keep your knees slightly bent.

•Raise your hands next to your ears and place your shoulders and arms flat against the wall while engaging your core.

•Push your arms up the wall above you while keeping them in contact with it.

•Repeat the movement by slowly lowering your arms.

•Repeat for a total of ten times.

7. Lunge with Hip Opener

This lunge with a hip opener movement is not your typical lunge. The lunge with a hip opener incorporates hip rotation and abduction rather than just knee and hip flexion and extension. This warm-up lunge is an active movement that helps build hip stability and prepares you for hinging movements like the squat and deadlift.

Try to make this movement as smooth and controlled as possible. With practice, this will become more fluid rather than in steps

Step-by-Step Instructions

•Stand tall and step forward with your right foot, leaving your left foot behind.

•Bend your right knee and lower your left leg almost to the floor as you lower your torso towards the floor.

•Slightly open your right knee by rotating it to the right. Keep your right foot firmly planted.

•Slightly open your left leg by slowly rotating it to the left. Hold for one count before returning to your starting position. Repeat on the other side.

•Experiment with 10 repetitions on each side.

8. Gate Opener

The gate opener exercise works your lower body, pelvis, and core muscles. This exercise improves hip mobility and range of motion while also building stability and balance. Warming up with the gate opener exercise will help prepare the psoas muscles, which run from your lower back region through your pelvis and to your femurs. These muscles help stabilise your back, and activating them during your warm-up will protect you from injury during hip-flexing exercises.

Step-by-Step Instructions

•Stand tall, feet hip-width apart, toes pointed forward or slightly outward.

•Keep your arms by your sides and your core engaged, pulling your shoulder blades back and down.

•Shift your weight to your right side and raise your left knee to about the height of your belly button. Move your right leg in and across your body's midline. Cross your left knee over your right leg.

•Next, extend your raised left leg to the left (abduction), opening your hip as far as possible. Maintain a strong core and forward-pointing hips.

•Return the knee to the centre slowly, then lower your foot to the ground to return to the starting position.
•Repeat on the other side.
•Complete 10 gate openers on each side.

9. Arm Circles with Reach
Shoulder joints are extremely mobile and easily injured. Many of us spend the majority of our days sitting and working in front of our computers, which causes our shoulders to become tense and weakened over time. Warming up the shoulders before a workout by dynamically moving the joints and tissues

is critical for preventing injury and activating the muscles.

Arm circles are a common warm-up exercise that you might have done in gym class. Adding a reach will help you increase your range of motion and warm up your shoulders even more.

Step-by-Step Instructions
•Stand tall and engage your core.
•Pay attention to your shoulders while slowly reaching your arm back behind you until you have to flip your arm around so your palm is facing forward.

•Reach as far back as possible while keeping your hips straight when reaching behind you and flipping your palm to face up.

•Flip your palm forward and extend your arm straight out in front of you. Reach forward again, attempting to increase your range of motion while keeping your core straight.

•Repeat 5 times, then reverse the motion for 5 more times.

•Repeat on the other side.

10. Prone Cobra

The prone cobra movement used during a warm-up is a yoga variation on the cobra pose. This is an isometric hold that is great for relieving back pain and preparing your body for thoracic and lumbar spine movements.

This is a corrective exercise that is especially beneficial before a workout after a long day at the office. Don't skip the thumbs-up motion with your palms facing outward if you want to get your shoulders into external rotation during this exercise.

Step-by-Step Instructions

•Lie on your stomach on the ground, hands by your sides, palms down.

•Lift your chest and torso as high as you can while keeping your chin tucked into your chest.

•To open your shoulders, lift your arms off the ground, thumbs pointing up to the ceiling. Your palms should be facing outward.

•Breathe through your nose and keep your shoulders open. If possible, hold for 30 seconds or longer. Build up to holding this pose for longer periods of time, up to 3 minutes at a time.

•Repeat the movement until you've held the contraction for 3 minutes total. If necessary, take breaks between sets.

Warming up is not just about getting your heart rate up. While this is important, it is even more important to start waking up your CNS, getting into the right mindset, and mobilising your joints to prepare you for the work ahead. When choosing your warm-up movements, stick with those that most closely mimic your training for the best results.

Chapter 2

Aerobic Fitness Essentials

This is where the magic happens in "Quick Workout for Beginners at Ease."

Why Aerobic Fitness Rocks:

Okay, let's keep it real. Aerobic exercise is like the superhero of workouts. It gets your heart pumping, boosts your stamina, and even gives your mood a high-five. We're talking about feeling good inside and out.

No Complications, Just Fun:

But hold up – we're not diving into some crazy, complicated routine. Nope. We've got simple aerobic moves that won't leave you huffing and puffing after one minute. Think brisk walking, maybe a bit of jogging in place – easy peasy.

Feel the Beat:

And guess what? You can do it to your favorite tunes. Throw on your go-to playlist, and let's turn this workout into a dance party. Who said exercise can't be a good time?

It's Your Time to Shine:

So, grab those sneakers, hit play on your favorite jams, and let's make aerobic fitness your new bestie. Chapter 2 is all about keeping it simple, effective, and heck, even a bit fun. Your exercise journey has just gotten a whole lot more exciting!

•Explanation of aerobic exercise and its benefits for overall health.

Aerobic exercise is a physical activity that works your body's vast muscle groups, is rhythmic and repetitive. It boosts your heart rate and how much oxygen your body uses. Examples of aerobic workouts include walking, cycling and swimming. It minimises the chances of heart disease, diabetes, high blood pressure and high cholesterol.

What is aerobic exercise?

Aerobic exercise is a physical activity that works big muscle groups in your body. This sort of workout is frequently rhythmic and repeated. You can control the intensity of your workout, which is how hard your body works during this sort of exercise.

Aerobic exercises boost your heart rate and how much oxygen your body requires. The term aerobic means "with oxygen." When you do aerobic exercise, your breathing controls the amount of oxygen that reaches your muscles to help you burn energy and move.

What is the distinction between aerobic and anaerobic training?
Aerobic and anaerobic are concepts that characterise how your body produces energy.

Aerobic means "with oxygen." When you participate in a continuous activity that elevates your heart rate, your cells use oxygen to make energy. An example of aerobic activity is walking.

Anaerobic implies "without oxygen." When you engage in a rapid, high-intensity activity, your cells aren't using oxygen to make energy. Stand by lifting is an illustration of anaerobic activity.

What are examples of aerobic exercises?
Aerobic exercises come in a variety of forms. Some of the most common include:
- Walking or jogging.

- Cycling.
- Cardio equipment.
- Swimming.

Walking or jogging

Walking is one of the most basic and widely available aerobic exercises. You can tailor the intensity to your level of fitness. Running is faster than jogging but slower than walking. Jogging is more strenuous on your joints than walking and should be avoided if you have an injury. This activity does not require any special equipment other than athletic shoes. You can walk almost anywhere, including malls, indoor tracks, and treadmills. This makes it simple to continue walking throughout the year. Walking is an excellent way to begin your first exercise programme.

Cycling

Cycling is an aerobic exercise that can be performed on either a stationary bike or a regular bicycle. You can increase the intensity of your workout by setting your stationary bike to a higher setting or riding on a route with more hills or inclines. Cycling may be ideal if you have arthritis or other joint-related conditions. This activity benefits your heart without causing the mechanical stress that walking does to your back, hips, knees, and ankles. When cycling outside, the weather may limit your activity.

Cardio Equipment

Cardio equipment consists of machines that raise your heart rate while you perform a repetitive motion. Some common types of cardio equipment are:
• A rowing machine.
• Stair climbers.
• An elliptical.
• A treadmill.
You can find these machines at your local gym or install one in your home. If you get one for at-home use, they're usually larger and can take

up a lot of space. Because there are so many different types of cardio machines, you should first try them out at a gym or fitness centre. It may take some time to determine which machine you prefer and which places less strain on areas of your body where you may have an injury or issue. Your healthcare provider can also advise you on the best type of cardio machine for you.

Swimming

Swimming is a low-impact activity in which you propel yourself through the water with your arms and legs. Swimming intensity increases more in open water than in a pool. If you have joint pain, water aerobics and water walking are good alternatives. The buoyancy provided by the water relieves joint stress. If you intend to swim or participate in water activities, make sure you do so under the supervision of a lifeguard in case of an emergency.

What are the benefits of aerobic exercise?
The benefits of aerobic exercise include:
• Building stronger bones.
• Enhancing muscle strength, endurance, and flexibility.
• Improving your balance.
Increasing your mental function.

• Assisting in weight management and/or weight loss.
• In addition, aerobic exercise can:
Reduce your chances of acquiring cardiovascular disease, hypertension, stroke, or diabetes.
• Improve your lung function.
• Lower your blood pressure.
• Increase HDL or "good" cholesterol.
• Help to better manage your blood sugar

What are the risks of aerobic exercises?
Physical activity can put you at danger of injury, which includes:
• Sprains and strains.
• Bone fracture.

- Joint pain.
- Muscle cramps.
- Pain or soreness.

How can I stay safe when conducting aerobic exercises?

Before beginning an exercise programme, consult with your healthcare physician. Inquire about any constraints you may have. If you have diabetes, hypertension, heart disease, arthritis, lung issues, or any other medical condition, you may require special exercise safety instructions. The sort of exercise you pick is a personal choice, but certain elements should be considered to lessen the chance of injury or complications and make exercise more enjoyable.

Injury prevention during aerobic activity
You can protect yourself from harm during aerobic activity by:
- Before beginning regular physical exercise, consult with your healthcare physician.
- Learning how to safely use workout equipment.
- Using proper technique and carrying out the workout as directed.
- Wearing the proper equipment or clothing.
- Being conscious of your environment.

- Stretching and warming up.

If you have unexpected shortness of breath, chest tightness, chest, shoulder, or jaw discomfort, lightheadedness, dizziness, confusion, or joint pain when exercising, you should stop immediately and call your healthcare professional.

Talking text:
Talking While executing the activity, attempt to carry on a conversation or communicate clearly. If speech is difficult, you may be engaging in a too strenuous activity. You can repeat this test

when your strength and stamina improve, and the results may alter.

How frequently should I perform aerobic exercises?

You should engage in 150 minutes of physical activity per week. The weekly amount equates to around 30 minutes per day, five days per week. This is the minimum recommendation for lowering your risk of heart disease, diabetes, hypertension, and high cholesterol.

It can be difficult to complete 150 minutes of aerobic activity every week. Follow these tips to make this amount of time simpler to complete: Make time in your day for physical activity.

Select activities that you enjoy.
It is excellent to exercise in little increments of
time, such as three 10-minute walks per day.
Engage in activities with friends or family.
Every day, you can do aerobic workouts. There
is no need to relax in between sessions unless
you are training at an intense level, such as for a
marathon, or if you have recurring joint
problems. If joint pain is a barrier, consult with
your doctor about less painful workouts.

How can I go about doing aerobic exercises?
Aerobic exercise should be performed in three
stages:

A period of preparation.
The exercise is progressing.
A period of rest.

Warming and cooling off

Every aerobic workout session should include a warmup and cooling time. Instead of static stretching, the warming period should consist of a gradual increase in the tempo and intensity of the exercise. This permits your body to enhance blood flow to your muscles, lowering your chances of injury to a muscle or joint. Warmup time should be between 5 and 10 minutes. The cooldown should last roughly the same length of time as the warmup, with the pace progressively dropping. Stretching activities would be beneficial following aerobic exercise.

Aerobic exercise progression

The amount of labour your body does throughout exercise should fluctuate as you progress or move to higher intensities. The progression of the activity should be determined by your tolerance and strength. If you're just getting started, you should take it slowly. You can gradually increase the amount of labour your body does throughout a workout if you're training for a marathon.

An aerobic workout can be advanced in three ways:

• Quicken your pace.
• Increase your resistance.
• Extend the period (time).

Any of these approaches, or a combination of them, will help you increase your aerobic fitness. The intensity should be gradually increased. You should only push yourself for a few minutes at a time.

Is it necessary for me to go to a gym to undertake aerobic exercises?

To undertake aerobic exercises, you do not need to go to a gym or fitness centre. At home, you can perform the following aerobic exercises:

- Go for a walk.
- Dancing is a skill.
- Riding a bicycle.
- Lawn mowing (with a push mower).

If you enjoy utilising specialised cardio equipment such as an elliptical or treadmill, you may prefer to undertake aerobic activities at a gym.

Aerobic exercises are a type of exercise that gets you up and moving. It raises your heart rate and causes you to sweat. Exercising can be difficult, but you can make it simpler by engaging in things you enjoy with people you enjoy spending time with. Before beginning a new physical activity, consult with your healthcare professional to ensure its safety. If you feel pain while exercising, stop immediately and call your clinician.

•Simple aerobic routines for beginners (e.g., brisk walking, jogging in place). Continue reading to learn more about aerobic workouts you may do at home or at the gym.

Remember to always with your doctor before starting a new aerobic exercise plan.

Aerobic workout at home

Home cardiovascular activities are possible. There are also numerous that require little to no equipment. Warm up for 5 to 10 minutes before beginning any exercise.

1. **Jump rope**

equipment includes gym shoes (sneakers) and a jump rope.

Benefit: Jumping rope helps to improve body awareness, hand-foot coordination, and agility.

Safety: Make sure your jump rope is suited to your height. Stand in the middle of the rope with

both feet and extend the handles to your armpits.
That is the height you intend to attain. To avoid
tripping on the rope, trim or tie it if it's too long.
Duration and frequency: 15–25 minutes, three to
five times a week
Following a jump rope circuit is a terrific indoor
or outdoor sport, but make sure you have enough
space. It should take you 15 to 25 minutes to
finish your circuit programme.
If you're just starting out:
Begin by running ahead while swinging the
jump rope over your head and beneath your feet.
Perform this movement for 15 seconds.

Next, reverse your direction and jog backward while swinging the jump rope. Perform this movement for 15 seconds.

Finish your set with a 15-second hopscotch jump. To perform this technique, jump rope in place and alternate between hopping your feet out to the sides and returning to the centre, like you would when doing jumping jacks. Perform this movement for 15 seconds.

Between sets, take a 15-second break.

Rep 18 times more.

If you're an intermediate exerciser, you can do the motions for 30 seconds each and rest for 30 seconds in between sets. The advanced circuit should be done for 60 seconds at a time, followed by a 60-second rest period.

2. Aerobic strength circuit

Equipment: shoes (sneakers), a firm chair or couch for dips

This exercise improves heart and cardiovascular health, boosts strength, and tones major muscle groups.

To avoid injury, focus on good form during each exercise. Maintain a reasonable heart rate throughout. During this practice, you should be able to hold a brief discussion.

Duration and frequency: 15–25 minutes, three to five times a week

This aerobic circuit is intended to raise your heart rate. For 1 minute, perform the following strength exercises:

Squats, lunges, pushups, triceps dips, and torso twists are examples of exercises. Then, for 1 minute of active rest, jog or march in place. This is a single circuit. Repeat the circuit 2–3 times more. You can take a 5-minute break between circuits. Following that, stretch lightly to relax.

3. Running or jogging

Equipment: running shoes

Benefits: Running is a highly effective kind of aerobic exercise. To name a few advantages, it can improve your heart health, burn fat and calories, and improve your mood.

Concerns about safety: Choose well-lit, populated running routes. Inform someone about your plans.

Duration and frequency: 20 to 30 minutes, twice a week. If you're just starting out, run for 20 to 30 minutes twice a week. During the run, keep your speed conversational. To begin, alternate 5 minutes of running and 1 minute of walking. Stretch after your run to avoid injuries.

4. Walking

Equipment: gym shoes (sneakers)

Benefits:

Walking every day can help lower your risk.Heart disease, obesity, diabetes, high blood pressure, and depression are all trusted sources. Walking in well-lit and populated locations is safer. To lessen your chance of injury, wear shoes with strong ankle support.
Duration and frequency: 150 minutes each week, or 30 minutes per day, five days a week
Aim for 150 minutes of walking each week if walking is your primary source of exercise. This can be divided into 30 minutes of walking five days a week. Alternatively, walk for 10 minutes at a time three times per day.
A fitness tracker can also be used to keep track of how many steps you take each day. If your

aim is to walk 10,000 steps per day, start with your baseline (the amount you already walk) and gradually increase your daily step count. You can accomplish this by increasing your daily steps by 500 to 1,000 steps every 1 to 2 weeks. So, once you've determined your starting point, add 500 to 1,000 steps. Then, one to two weeks later, boost your daily step count by 500 to 1,000 steps.

Aerobic workouts in the gym

A good place to do some cardio exercise is at your local gym. They most likely have treadmills, stationary cycles, and elliptical machines. There may also be a pool where you may swim laps.

If you are unsure how to utilise a piece of exercise equipment, always seek the advice of a professional or trainer.

5. Swimming

Equipment: pool, swimsuit, goggles (optional)
Benefits:
Swimming is a low-impact exercise that is beneficial for persons who are prone to or recovering from injuries, as well as those who have limited mobility. It is a good choice if you are prone to injury because it is a low-impact workout. You're also boosting your heart rate, muscle strength, and endurance without placing any more strain on your body.

Swimming alone should be avoided, and if possible, find a pool with a lifeguard on duty. If you're new to swimming, start with swim lessons. Duration and frequency: 2 to 5 times per week, 10 to 30 minutes. To extend your duration, add 5 minutes to your swim time each week.
Try swimming as aerobic workout if your gym offers a pool. It is a good choice if you are prone to injury because it is a low-impact workout. You're also boosting your heart rate, muscle strength, and endurance without placing any more strain on your body.
You can begin by swimming laps with a single stroke, such as freestyle. Add more strokes as you swim more. For instance, you could swim

one to four laps of freestyle followed by one to four laps of breaststroke or backstroke. Rest on the pool's edge between laps if you grow fatigued. Always observe the pool's safety rules and guidelines when swimming.

6. Stationary bike

Equipment: stationary bike
Benefits:
This low-impact workout can assist in the development of leg strength and cardiovascular endurance.
Ask a trainer at the gym for assistance in setting the bike so that the seat is at the proper height.

This will help lower your chances of getting hurt or falling off your bike.

When biking at home, a common rule is to adjust the bike seat height so that your knee has a 5- to 10-degree bend (slight bend) before achieving full extension. This relieves compression on your knee joint. It is not advisable to fully extend your knee while riding a stationary bike.

Duration and frequency: 35-45 minutes, three times a week

Another low-impact fitness alternative is to ride a stationary bike. Stationary bikes provide a good aerobic workout, help with leg strength development, and are simple to use. Cycling classes on stationary cycles are available at many gyms and training studios. You can, however, benefit from a stationary bike workout even if you are not enrolled in a class.

After stretching and warming up for 5 to 10 minutes by cycling at an easy rhythm, raise your tempo to 75 to 80 rotations per minute (RPM) and aim for 20 to 30 minutes of consistent cycling. Allow for a 5-minute cooling period. Finish with a stretch.

Maintain enough resistance on the bike so that you feel like you're pushing the pedals rather than the pedals pushing your feet. To make the workout more tough, increase the resistance.

7. Elliptical

Equipment: elliptical machine

Benefits:

Elliptical machines provide a terrific aerobic workout that is less taxing on the knees, hips, and back than running on the road or trails.

Look up, not down, for safety. Use the handles to help you get on and off the machine if you feel wobbly.

Duration and frequency: 20 to 30 minutes, twice a week.

The elliptical machine may appear frightening at first, but once you get the hang of it, it's very simple to use. After warming up for 5 to 10 minutes, keep your posture upright while

moving the machine with your legs in a pedal motion. Look ahead the entire time rather than down at your feet. Keep your spine straight and your abdominal muscles engaged. Exit the machine and stretch or cool down.
Increase the resistance on the machine to make the workout more difficult.

Aerobic class workouts

If you dislike working out alone, a class can offer a helpful and encouraging setting. If you're new, ask the instructor to demonstrate proper form. If you're a newbie, they can help you alter the exercises if necessary.

To begin, attend group courses at your local fitness centre two to three times per week. If you enjoy the workout, you can always go more frequently later on.

8. Cardio kickboxing

Equipment: gym shoes (sneakers)
Benefits:
Kickboxing is a high-impact workout that improves strength and endurance. It may also help to relieve tension and improve reflexes. Drink plenty of water throughout the class for your own safety. Take a pause if you feel dizzy. Duration and frequency: 60 minutes per week, one to three times per week

Cardio kickboxing is a martial arts, boxing, and aerobics hybrid. Your lesson may begin with a warmup that includes running, jumping jacks, or strengthening exercises like pushups. The main workout will then consist of a sequence of punches, kicks, and hand strikes.
At the end, there may be core or strengthening exercises. Always end your workout with a stretch and cool down.

9. Zumba

Equipment: gym shoes (sneakers)
Benefits: Zumba is good for your heart, it improves coordination, it tones your entire body, and it may help you relax.

Drink plenty of water during the class for your own safety. If you feel fatigued or dizzy, take a rest. If you are prone to ankle injuries, you should wear shoes with strong ankle support. Duration and frequency: 60 minutes per week, one to three times per week

Zumba is an excellent cardio workout if you enjoy dancing. After warming up, your instructor will lead the class in simple dancing moves matched to exciting music. After that, you'll stretch and cool down.

It is necessary to wear shoes. Drink plenty of water during class. If you grow fatigued, you may always take a break and rejoin.

10. Indoor cycling class

Equipment: stationary bike, cycling shoes (optional), padded bicycle shorts or pants (optional)

Benefits:

Indoor cycling classes increase strength, muscle tone, and cardiovascular endurance.

If you're new or need a refresher, ask the instructor to assist you with setting up the stationary bike. Reduce your resistance if you become exhausted, and take a break if you become lightheaded.

Duration and frequency: 45 to 60 minutes, once or twice a week.

A cycle class, as opposed to a leisurely bike ride, will raise your heart rate. For optimal training effects, it may contain resistance and climb (incline) parts. This will assist you in increasing your strength and toning your muscles. Some lessons necessitate the use of cycling shoes that "clip" into the bike.. These are normally available for hire at your facility.

The majority of lessons are 45 to 60 minutes and include a warm-up, cool-down, and stretch.

Bring water to class with you. If you're just starting out, you can lower the resistance on your bike and cycle lightly for a break if you get fatigued.

Chapter 3

Strength Training Basics

We're diving into the muscle-building world in "Quick Workout for Beginners at Ease."
Why Strength Training is the Bomb:
Let's get one thing straight – you don't need to become a bodybuilder. But adding a bit of strength training? Oh, that's like giving your muscles a little pep talk. It tones you up, revs up that metabolism, and just makes you feel strong and awesome.
No Fancy Equipment, No Problem:

And here's the beauty – you don't need a gym full of fancy gear. We're talking bodyweight exercises that you can do anywhere. Squats, push-ups – simple stuff that packs a punch.

Start Slow, Build Strong:

Now, don't stress about lifting heavy right out of the gate. We're easing into this. A few sets of squats, some push-ups – trust me, you'll feel the burn, but in a good way.

You Got This:

So, grab a water bottle (or a couple of soup cans, no judgment), and let's make strength training your new favorite thing. Chapter 3 is all about keeping it real, keeping it simple, and getting you stronger, one rep at a time!

•Importance of strength training for muscle tone and metabolism.

Every fitness regimen should involve strength training, and stronger muscles are just one of the health benefits.

Strength training can help with bone health, making aerobic exercise more productive, reducing injury, and promoting healthy ageing.

Wouldn't you want to start exercising if you knew it could assist your heart, improve your balance, strengthen your bones and muscles, and help you lose or maintain weight? Strength exercise, according to research, can provide all of these benefits and more.

According to the National Academy of Sports Medicine (NASM), strength training, also known as weight or resistance training, is a physical activity designed to improve muscular strength and fitness by exercising a specific muscle or muscle group against external resistance, such as free weights, weight machines, or your own body weight.
"The basic principle is to apply a load and overload the muscle so that it needs to adapt and get stronger," says Neal Pire, CSCS, an ACSM-certified exercise physiologist and executive director of the Greater New York ACSM regional organisation. What everyone should know is that strength training isn't just for bodybuilders and professional athletes. "Strength training is critical, not just for looking good and being strong, but also for preventing diseases of ageing," says Gabrielle Lyon, DO, a

functional medicine practitioner in New York City and founder of the Institute for Muscle-Centric Medicine, a functional medicine practice.

According to the Cleveland Clinic, regular strength or resistance training is beneficial for people of all ages and fitness levels in order to help avoid the natural loss of lean muscle mass that occurs with ageing (the medical name for this loss is sarcopenia). According to a 2019 research review, it can also benefit those with chronic health issues such as obesity, diabetes, or heart disease.

Strength training may possibly extend your life: A meta-analysis released in February 2022 discovered that persons who engage in weight training are less likely to die prematurely than those who do not, even if aerobic exercise is not part of their regimen.

Strength training is fundamentally based on functional movements — lifting, pushing, pulling — to build muscle and coordination required for daily activities, according to Ramona Braganza, a Los Angeles-based celebrity personal trainer certified by the Canadian fitness education organisation Canfitpro.

"While the term "strength training" may be intimidating to some, it improves your ability to move in a safe and efficient manner throughout your lifetime," she continued. For instance, your capacity to lift something and place it on a shelf, carry groceries in the door, bend down and pick something up, or rise up after falling down. "Getting up off the floor requires you to recruit muscles in your upper body, abs, legs, and glutes," Braganza said.

The U.S. Department of Health and Human Services (HHS) recommends that children and adolescents ages 6 to 17 integrate some strength training within their daily 60 minutes of physical activity three days per week. Adults should try to conduct at least two days per week of moderate or vigorous muscle-strengthening workouts that target all muscle groups.

You should also recover in between strength training sessions.

Pire said, "You don't get better when you work out; you get better between workouts"

"You should give yourself a day in between strength training to allow your body to recover and rebuild the muscle tissue from the stimulus of lifting or resistance."

Strength Training Can Help Your Health in 8 Ways

Aside from the well-publicized (and constantly Instagrammed) benefit of increasing muscular tone and definition, how can strength training help? Here are just a few examples of the numerous possibilities:

1. Strength training improves your strength and fitness.

This is the most obvious benefit, but it should not be underestimated. "Muscle strength is crucial in making it easier to do the things you need to do on a day-to-day basis," Pire explains, especially as we age and inevitably lose muscle.

Strength training, often known as resistance training, entails contracting your muscles against an opposing force in order to strengthen and tone them.

Resistance training is classified into two kinds, according to the Encyclopaedia of Behavioural Medicine:

• **Isometric Strength** This entails tightening your muscles against a stationary object, such as the floor in a pushup.

•**Isotonic Resistance** Training As in weight lifting, this includes tightening your muscles across a range of motion.

2. Strength exercise promotes bone health and muscle mass.

According to Harvard Health Publishing, we begin losing 3 to 5 percent of our lean muscle mass per decade around the age of 30.

A 2017 study found that 30 minutes twice a week of high-intensity resistance and impact training improved functional performance, as well as bone density, structure, and strength in postmenopausal women with low bone mass – with no side consequences.

Similarly, the HHS physical activity guidelines state that muscle-strengthening activities help everyone maintain or improve muscular mass, strength, and power, all of which are important for bone, joint, and muscle health as we age.

3. Strength training aids in the efficient burning of calories. All forms of exercise help to increase your metabolism (the rate at which your resting body burns calories throughout the day).

Your body continues to burn calories after strength training as it returns to a more rested condition (in terms of energy expended) with both aerobic activity and strength training. According to the American Council on Exercise (ACE), this is a process known as "excess post-exercise oxygen consumption." When you conduct strength, weight, or resistance training, your body wants more energy based on how much energy you're exerting (the more energy is demanded, the harder you work). So, depending on how much energy you put into the workout, you can amp up the result. That implies more calories burned during the workout, as well as more calories burned afterward as your body recovers to a resting state.

4. Long-term weight loss is aided by strength training.

Because strength training increases extra post-exercise oxygen consumption more than aerobic exercise, it can help exercisers lose weight faster than aerobic exercise alone, according to Pire. "[Resistance or strengthening exercise] keeps your metabolism active after exercising much longer than after an aerobic workout."

This is because lean tissue is more active tissue in general. "If you have more muscle mass, you'll burn more calories — even in your sleep — than if you didn't have that extra lean body mass," he said.

A 2017 study found that dieters who did strength training exercises four times a week for 18 months lost the most fat (about 18 pounds, compared to 10 pounds for nonexercisers and 16 pounds for aerobic exercisers) when compared to dieters who did not exercise or only aerobic exercise.

You may even be able to lose even more body fat if you mix strength training with calorie restriction. A short study published in 2018 indicated that people who followed a combined full-body resistance exercise and diet for four months reduced their fat mass while enhancing lean muscle mass more than either resistance training or dieting alone.

5. Strength Training Aids in the Development of Better Body Mechanics

According to previous study, strength exercise improves your balance, coordination, and posture. One 2017 study found that doing at least one resistance training session per week — either alone or as part of a programme with a variety of workouts — resulted in a 37 percent increase in muscle strength, a 7.5 percent increase in muscle mass, and a 58 percent increase in functional capacity (linked to fall risk) in frail, elderly adults.

Increasing walking speed may reduce the risk of diabetes.

"Balance is dependent on the strength of the muscles that keep you on your feet," Pire said. "The stronger those muscles, the better your balance."

6. Strength training can aid in the management (and prevention) of chronic diseases.
Strength training has been shown in studies to aid persons with a variety of chronic diseases, including neuromuscular disorders, HIV, chronic obstructive pulmonary disease, and various malignancies. Strength training, along with other healthy lifestyle modifications, can assist improve glucose control in the more than 30 million Americans with type 2 diabetes, according to the Centres for Disease Control and Prevention and a 2017 study. Furthermore, according to a 2019 review published in Frontiers in Physiology, frequent resistance

exercise can help avoid chronic mobility issues, heart disease, type 2 diabetes, and cancer.

7. Strength exercise boosts energy and elevates mood.

Strength training has been validated as a viable therapy option (or add-on treatment) for depression symptoms in a meta-analysis of 33 clinical trials published in 2018.

"All exercise boosts mood because it increases endorphins," says Pire. However, he claims that a new study into neurochemical and neuromuscular adaptations to strength training gives additional evidence that it has a positive effect on the brain.

A 2019 study also found evidence that strength training may help you sleep better. And we all know that obtaining a good night's sleep can help you maintain a positive attitude.

It has been demonstrated that strength training improves cardiovascular health.
According to the HHS, muscle-strengthening activities, in addition to aerobic exercise, help to improve blood pressure and reduce the risk of hypertension and heart disease. A systematic review of 38 randomised controlled trials published in 2021 found that weight training combined with aerobic exercise is more effective than aerobic exercise alone in heart disease rehabilitation.

8. Strength training has been shown to improve cardiovascular health.

Muscle-strengthening activities, in addition to aerobic exercise, assist improve blood pressure and minimise the risk of hypertension and heart disease, according to the HHS. A systematic evaluation of 38 randomised controlled studies published in 2021 showed that weight training mixed with aerobic exercise is more effective in heart disease rehabilitation than aerobic exercise alone.

•Bodyweight exercises for beginners (e.g., squats, push-ups).

Think you can't do a good exercise or grow muscle with your own body weight? Think again. Getting fit doesn't have to be complicated. Keep it simple, safe, and effective with bodyweight workouts you can do anytime and anywhere for the rest of your life.

Whether you are an athlete, a leisure workout enthusiast, or someone who has never lifted anything more than a small child or daily household object, utilising your body weight as resistance is one of the finest methods to get and stay in shape for years to come.

Benefits of Bodyweight Exercises

Here are 12 advantages of working out that will encourage and thrill you.

1. It helps improve any muscle imbalances, especially from rounded shoulders and tight hips from sitting too long (hello, new work from the home model).

2. It works the whole body.

3. It lays down an excellent foundation for future weighted programming.

4. It helps improve strength, endurance, balance, flexibility, and coordination.

5. It can increase your confidence.

6. It saves time going to the gym.

7. It can be done anywhere, so there is never an excuse not to work out.

8. No equipment is necessary.

9. It never gets boring.

10. It's free.

11. It's great for any body type.

Will I Be Able to Build Muscles Using Only My Body Weight?

Yes!! Muscle fibres break down after an intense workout and must be repaired. Muscles will strengthen and expand throughout this mending phase. It is important to note that for this process to take place, the body must be pushed beyond of its comfort zone. External resistance, like as free weights, barbells, or bands, will speed up this process and is an excellent complement to any strength programme, but it is possible to achieve the same results with only your body weight.

The trick is to keep altering your training variables (sets, reps, intensity, time under tension) as you develop. Once you've learned your technique, it's time to take it to the next level by alternating between high-intensity and slow-paced workouts, focusing on activating the muscle during the contraction phase, as I demonstrate in the video.

To get you started, let's break down a few basic workouts and body sections.

To begin, the body can do seven basic movements: pushing, pulling, hinge, squatting, twisting, skipping, and leaping. From these seven, there are numerous variations for each body area, which I will demonstrate below. Bodyweight workouts train all of your muscles, including your heart, while increasing your endurance.

1. Plank Push-Ups and Back Extensions
2. Chest - Push-ups, Regular Incline, High to Low Plank
3. Arms - Side Plank Hip Drop, Side Plank Hip Drop, Dips
4. Core/Hips - Planks (high and low; can be done from the kitchen counter), Elevated Mountain Climbers, Opposite Arm Leg Reach, Bear Crawl Hold, Isometric Knee Press (Single and Double Knee Hold), Heel Drops (Single and Double Heel Drop), Deadbug, Crunches, Floor Bridge

5. Legs and Hips
6. Seated Bent Knee Extensions and Seated Straight Leg Lifts for the Quadriceps
7. Side leg raises, deadlifts, prone leg lifts, and glute extensions are all examples of hip exercises.
8. Chair Squat, Step Out Squat, Plie Squat, and Wall Squat Hold
9. Step-ups, stationary lunges, side lunges, curtsy lunges, and swing lunges are all examples of lunges.

Creating a Bodyweight Exercise Programme
The variety of bodyweight workouts is limitless and can be applied to any current living

circumstance. Use the basic structure below to keep your muscles wondering whether you have 10 minutes or an hour. If you're just getting started, start with 20 minutes twice a week for two to four weeks. Increase the duration and number of days per week as your fitness level improves.

The best part about bodyweight workouts is that there are so many different versions that you will never get bored. Choose one exercise from each category. Always begin with a movement that works multiple muscles at once, such as push-ups and squats, and then progress to exercises that work smaller muscles, such as dips for the triceps.

1. Plank Push-Ups

• Begin on your elbows on a raised surface, such as a kitchen counter or dining table.

• Take a step back and together with your feet, supporting your body weight on your elbows.

• Maintain a straight line from your head to your toes.

• Brace your core by pushing your stomach muscles in towards the rear of your body and begin to retract your shoulder blades as if squeezing a pencil, then push the counter away with your core and elbows and return to the beginning position.

• Carry out the required number of repetitions (reps).
• Your entire body should move in unison.

2. Push-Ups
• Begin by placing your hands shoulder-width apart on a raised surface, such as a kitchen counter or dining table.
• Step your feet back and together, supporting your whole weight on your hands and keeping a straight line from your head to your toes.
• Brace your core by pushing your stomach muscles in towards the rear of your body, then bend your elbows and drop your chest towards

the counter, then straighten your arms and push back up to the beginning position.
• Complete the number of reps specified.
• Your entire body should move in unison.

3. Step-Out Squat
• Begin by putting your feet together.
• Take a step to the right and descend your hips behind you, pushing through your heels. • •
Keep your knees behind your toes.
• Stand up and take a step together, tucking your tailbone under and clenching your buttocks at the top.
• Complete the prescribed reps.
• Repeat on the other side.

4. Stationary Lunge

• Take a step out around hip bone/hip distance.
• Take a step back with your right foot and stagger your stance around the length of your leg.
• Lift your back heel off the ground and begin to bend your legs, lowering your body to the floor.
• Make sure to put more weight into your front heel and keep your front knee behind your toes.
• Complete the prescribed reps.

5. The Hip Bridge

• Lie on your back on the floor or on a couch.
• Kneel down and place your feet on the floor.

• Squeeze your buttocks and press your hips to the sky as you press through your feet.
• Lower halfway down, then repeat.
• Complete the prescribed reps.

6. Isometric Knee Press

Start with one side at a time or both legs on a tabletop, depending on your core strength.

LEVEL ONE: SINGLE-LEG KNEE PRESSURE

• Lie on your back on the floor or on a couch.
• Kneel down and place your right foot on the floor.

• While keeping the left knee bent, raise it off the floor to a 90° angle (also known as tabletop position).
• Place your left hand on your left thigh.
• Push your hand into your thigh and your thigh into your hand at the same moment. Your abdominal muscles should tense.
• Hold that contraction for 10 seconds before pausing.
• Complete the prescribed reps.
• Change sides.

DOUBLE KNEE PRESS (LEVEL 2)

• The same format as before, except this time both legs will be in tabletop position.
• Brace the abdominals for 10 seconds, then pause.
• Complete the number of reps specified.

Begin with bodyweight workouts if your objective is to move and feel better in your body while progressing to an advanced fitness level. It will not only lay a firm foundation, but it will also help you avoid injury and give you the confidence to continue going to more difficult activities.

By including bodyweight workouts into your weekly routine, you can commit to yourself and future strength increases. I guarantee you won't be sorry.

Chapter 4

Core Exercise Fundamentals

Fundamentals of Core Training examines how to define the core, identify its anatomical components, and comprehend how each component contributes to the stabilisation and mobilisation of the lumbar-pelvic-hip complex. You use your core to perform many everyday tasks, such as pulling a grocery cart or putting on shoes. It also has an impact on your balance, posture, and stability.

Contrary to popular opinion, your core muscles do not only consist of your abdominal muscles.

Muscles in your back and surrounding your pelvis are also included.

Your core, or trunk, consists of your:
 Erector spinae is a type of spinae. The erector spinae is a back muscle that runs up the spine. It enables you to stand up straight after leaning over, bend sideways, and rotate your head.
 Rectus abdominis is an abdominis muscle. The rectus abdominis abdominal muscle is used when you bend forward. It's also referred to as the "six pack" muscle.
 Obliques. Your internal and external oblique muscles assist you in rotating or bending your trunk.

The transverse abdominis muscle. Your pelvis is stabilised by the transverse abdominis, which wraps across the front and side of your trunk.
 Multifidus. Your spine is supported by the multifidus in your back.
Your core muscles also include the following:
- pelvic floor
- diaphragm
- gluteus maximus

hamstrings, hip flexors, and hip adductors)
Keeping these muscles strong helps stabilise your body, support your spine, and improve your overall fitness.

•Understanding the core muscles and their role.

When most people think about core strength, they think about an abdominal six-pack. While it and improving performance. Having a strong or stable core can often prevent overuse injuries, and can help boost resiliency and ease of rehab from acute injury. The core also includes the pelvic floor musculature, and maintaining core stability looks good, this toned outer layer of abdominal musculature is not the same as a strong core.

What is the "core" and why is core strength so important?

The core is a group of muscles that stabilizes and controls the pelvis and spine (and therefore influences the legs and upper body). Core strength is less about power and more about the subtleties of being able to maintain the body in ideal postures — to unload the joints and promote ease of movement. For the average person, this helps them maintain the ability to get on and off the floor to play with their children or grandchildren, stand up from a chair, sit comfortably at a desk, or vacuum and rake without pain. For athletes, it promotes more efficient movement, therefore preventing injury can help treat and prevent certain types of incontinence.

The problem with a weak core

As we age, we develop degenerative changes, very often in the spine. The structures of the bones and cartilage are subject to wear and tear. Very often, we are able to completely control and eliminate symptoms with the appropriate core exercises. Having strong and stable postural muscles helps suspend the bones and other structures, allowing them to move better. Scoliosis, a curving or rotation of the spine, can also often be controlled with the correct postural exercises. Having an imbalanced core can lead to problems up and down the body. Knee pain is often caused by insufficient pelvic stabilization. Some runners develop neck and back pain when running because the "shock absorbers" in their core could use some work.

Finding the right core strengthening program for you

A good core program relies less on mindless repetition of exercise and focuses more on awareness. People with good core strength learn to identify and activate the muscles needed to accomplish the task. Learning to activate the core requires concentration, and leads to being more in tune with the body.

There is no one method of core strengthening that works for everyone. Some people do well with classes (though it can be easy do the repetitions without truly understanding the targeted muscle groups). Others use Pilates or yoga to discover where their core is. Physical therapists are excellent resources, as they can provide one-on-one instruction and find a method that works for any person with any background at any ability level. It sometimes takes patience for people to "find" their core, but once they do, it can be engaged and activated during any activity — including walking, driving, and sitting. While building the core starts with awareness and control, athletes can further challenge their stability with more complex movements that can be guided by athletic trainers and other fitness specialists. Daily practice of core engagement can lead to healthier movement patterns that allow for increased mobility and independence throughout the course of our lives.

What Is Core Stability?

Core stability refers to the way our core muscles help keep our spine straight and stable as we do everyday tasks. These muscles allow us to sit, stand, walk, and do things like shovel snow without pain.

For those who are physically active, core stability also helps prevent injuries due to overuse of muscles. A strong core can make movements smoother and more effective, thereby reducing the likelihood of injury and improving your performance and skill.

Core strength affects more than just posture, though. Your core includes your pelvis, and these muscles can help prevent incontinence. Weakness in the core can lead to pain and issues all over your body such as the back, neck, and joints like the knees. Your core muscles naturally weaken as you age, but sitting for long periods of time can cause core weakness as well. Luckily, there are many exercises you can try to help strengthen your core muscles.

•Beginner-friendly core exercises (e.g., plank, bicycle crunches).

How to Strengthen Your Core

There are a wide range of activities you can attempt to assist with fortifying your center muscles. Some exercises involve further movement, while others incorporate static holds. These types of exercises generally work stylish on a coated bottom or exercise mat. You may find some types of exercises work better for you than others.

Abdominal crunch. The stomach crunch is a work of art, well known choice for reinforcing center muscles. To do this move:

- Lie level on your back on a strong surface.
- Either twist your knees so that the lower portion of your feet are level with the floor, or position the bottoms of your feet against a wall and curve your knees 90 degrees.
- Utilize your stomach muscles to pull your head and shoulders off the floor.
- To try not to strain your neck, fold your arms over your chest and keep your eyes on the roof.
- Hold the muscle constriction at the top for three full breaths.
- Get back to your beginning position and rehash.

Bridge.
The scaffold is an extraordinary method for working various muscles all at once. To do this move:

• Lie level on your back with your knees twisted.

• Push through the bottoms of your feet to lift your hips off the floor. Make an effort not to curve your back or press it into the floor.

• Hold here for three full breaths.

• Get back to your beginning position and rehash

Forward plank. A board is a static hold move that prepares a few center muscles. To do a customary forward board:

• Get into a customary pushup position with your elbows straightforwardly under your shoulders, your pelvis shifted somewhat forward, and your center, back, and hindquarters held tight. Your feet ought to be together.

• Try not to let your back and hips hang or curve.

• Stand firm on this foothold for however long you are agreeable.

• On the off chance that a customary board is excessively troublesome, you can change this activity by laying on your elbows rather than the centers of your hands or kneeling down rather than your feet. Fledglings might pick to do both.

Side plank.

A side plank is another type of plank. It, like the standard plank, can be adjusted to make the exercise easier or more difficult.To do a side plank, do the following:

• Lie down on your side. Balance yourself on the forearm of your lower arm. If you're lying on your left side, this is your left arm; if you're resting on your right side, this is your right arm. Your elbow should be 90 degrees bent and directly under your shoulder.

• Raise your hips off the ground and contract your abs. Weight should be distributed evenly between your elbow and your feet/ankles. Lift your hips high enough to keep a straight line. should be split between your elbow and your feet/ankles. Lift your hips high enough to keep a straight line.

Maintain this position for as long as you are at ease.

Bend your lower leg and place your weight on your knee and leg rather than your foot and ankle to make this manoeuvre easier. To make it more difficult, straighten your arm and balance on your palm rather than your elbow.

Superman. The superman is an exercise that targets your back muscles specifically. To execute this manoeuvre:

• Lie down on your stomach, arms and legs extended.

• Raise one arm off the ground, keeping it straight, and hold for three breaths.

• Return to the beginning position and do the same with the opposite arm.
• Raise one leg straight off the floor and hold for three deep breaths.
• Return to your starting position and do the opposite side.
• To make this motion more challenging, raise one arm and the opposing leg at the same moment, then swap.

Chapter 5

Balancing Act.

Balance is more than your capacity to stay upright and properly distribute your weight as you move steadily; it is an anchor for your well-being and is sometimes taken for granted until it is damaged.

A strong sense of balance helps you react quickly and maintain equilibrium while crossing uneven terrain on a beach walk or engaging in sports, lowering the chance of slips, trips, and falls. To completely comprehend balance, we will look at the combination of sensorimotor controls that our bodies use for balance, as well as symptoms and circumstances of imbalance that may necessitate medical attention and even physical treatment.

We invite you to use our simple assessments of essential at-home exercises to access and improve your balance, and to learn why functional fitness is an ideal alternative for maintaining and boosting stability.

For more complex imbalance symptoms or situations, a doctor's assessment is advised. Please discontinue self-assessment and at-home activities if you experience unsteadiness, dizziness, lightheadedness, blurred vision, falling, disorientation, room spinning, or the sensation of moving when stationary.

Putting Your Balance to the Test

While a tightrope or balance beam are superior balance indicators, these basic exams can provide a picture of your current balance. A few basic tests might help you assess your balance and identify areas for improvement:

Note: We recommend testing with a trusted friend, standing near a sturdy object to stop yourself if you become imbalanced, and consulting with your doctor about your postural stability problems.

Romberg Test:
Stand with your arms folded in front of you or straight out in front of you, both feet touching and facing forward. Rep with your eyes closed. Visit your doctor or have a friend monitor your stance for one minute and record any motions, such as swaying.

Single-Legged Stance Test (SLST): Stand on one leg for as long as you can and see how long you can keep your balance. Hold for one minute and then repeat on the opposite leg for three sets.

Advanced SLST: Stand on one leg with your eyes closed for 30 seconds or as long as you can under supervision.

Straight Line: Walk in a straight line from heel to toe, as if you were taking a sobriety test. You can make it more difficult by stepping on a 24 board or other sturdy item.

Understanding Sensorimotor Controls in Balance

Every movement, touch, or vibration detected by your body transmits impulses to your brain via the dorsal column, the central nervous system's (brain and spinal cord) pathway, via sensory receptors in your skin, joints, and muscles that detect motion and position. Proprioception occurs when your brain combines sensations with data from other systems, such as your inner ear's vestibular system and vision, to understand your body's location in respect to the environment. By removing eyesight during the balancing test, your doctor can assess the function of your dorsal column.

Physical Therapy Can Assist You in Finding Your Balance

Medical treatments like Symbios physical therapy can help you regain your balance after an injury, a health condition, eyesight problems, certain drugs, or ageing. Physical therapists are educated to analyse individual needs and create customised exercise programmes that address specific areas of weakness or imbalance. To improve overall stability, these programmes may incorporate a combination of strength training, flexibility exercises, and coordination drills. Furthermore, physical therapists can advise on good body mechanics and provide solutions for improving balance in daily activities.

Valuable Balance Exercises You Can Do at Home

Include these exercises in your workout plan to improve your balance, stability, and overall functional fitness. Listen to your body, start cautiously, and advance progressively, as with fitness programme. If you have any concerns or pre-existing health conditions, speak with Symbios Health or a licenced fitness specialist before beginning a new workout plan.

Flamingo Stance

Start with standing on one leg, knee slightly bent. Lift the opposing foot off the ground, bringing the sole of your foot to the inner of the calf or thigh of your standing leg (at a comfortable level for you). To aid in balance, locate a focus point in front of you. Hold the position for 20-30 seconds before rotating to the opposite leg. To enhance difficulty, try closing your eyes or incorporating tiny motions such as lifting your arms.

Tandem Knee Lift Stance

Stand in a straight line, with the heel of one foot directly in front of the toes of the other. Maintain your focus and engage your core. Maintaining the tandem stance, lift your back leg towards your chest. Hold the raised knee for a moment before lowering it. Repeat this movement on one leg for 10-15 times before moving to the other. This workout tests your balance and improves hip stability.

Balance on One Leg with Your Eyes Closed
Stand on one leg, marginally bowed at the knee.
Close your eyes and concentrate on keeping your
balance once you feel stable. Keep your hips
level and your core engaged. Hold the position
for 20-30 seconds before transferring to the
opposite leg. This exercise tests your
proprioception (awareness of your body in
space) and improves the muscles that stabilise
your ankles, knees, and hips.

Standing on One Leg
To begin, sit in a firm chair with your feet flat on
the floor. Transfer your weight to one leg and
elevate the opposing foot off the ground slightly.
Stand up from the chair using only one leg. Once

you're up, slowly lower yourself back to a seated posture. Repeat this movement on one leg for 10-12 reps before moving to the other. This workout improves your balance while also strengthening your hips, thighs, and lower back.

How Functional Fitness Helps with Balance
Functional fitness focuses on workouts that mirror real-life movements, improving your ability to do daily tasks efficiently while avoiding injuries. This method immediately helps to improved balance by activating different muscle groups at the same time. Squats, lunges, and stability ball routines can assist strengthen the core and lower body as well as stabilise

muscles, which are important for maintaining balance. The skilled training experts at SymbiosFIT would love to work with you to improve technique and ensure appropriate form during workouts for faster results.

Symbios urges you to put balance first in your fitness quest and reap the benefits of a more steady and injury-resistant lifestyle. Regular self-evaluation, functional exercises, and, if necessary, the expertise of physical therapists can all play important roles in ensuring that your balance stays a firm foundation for overall well-being.

•The significance of balancing exercise for stability.

What Is the Importance of Balance Training?
Your balance training is beneficial not only to your balance, but also to a variety of other areas. Balance training can help ensure that you are performing activities correctly while also reducing your chance of injury.
It's an excellent technique to enhance your balance, coordination, agility, and strength without overworking your joints or muscles.

What is the significance of balance training?
This book will cover the importance of balance

training and why it should be incorporated in any workout plan!

What exactly is balancing training, and why do I require it?

Balance is something we all use on a daily basis, but have you ever considered how it works?
You might be shocked by all of this - the neurological system and your eyes, for example, both contribute to balance.
Age, muscle strength/endurance, joint range of motion (particularly in the ankles), weight-bearing activity, and other factors all contribute to improved balance.

Balance training can help improve some or all of the factors required for proper posture and balance. It is significant because it aids in the prevention of falls, which are most common in adults over the age of 60.

Balance routines will keep you feeling younger than your actual age if you're young at heart. Balance training can help you and everyone in your family stay safe, no matter who you are.

What is the process of balance training?
Using balance tools is an excellent approach to train your body in the same area where it will be utilised without fear of falling! Using stability

ball, balancing cushions/boards, or even skateboards if you have one lying around...?

Increases Reaction Time

Balance exercise enhances response time, or the capacity to respond fast and precisely.

This means that by strengthening your balance, you can be faster at catching a ball or changing direction in sports.

Perfecting this talent will provide you an advantage over others - reaction speed has been shown to diminish with age, but it does not have to.

Balance training helps younger athletes increase their reaction speeds, while it also helps elderly folks maintain their reactive abilities.

Increases strength

Balance training causes the body to use more muscle fibres, increasing power and endurance while also improving coordination, agility, balance, and speed.

Balance training is vital for overall physical health regardless of how frequently or what type of workouts you undertake.

When balancing on an unsteady surface, your core muscles must be activated at all times in order to maintain stability.

This builds a stronger foundation for mobility by strengthening your abdominal and back muscles (rather than just activating these muscles during crunches).
As a result, there is less danger of injury during workouts and overall performance improves. Balance training also helps activate your glutes and inner thigh muscles, which can help you avoid knee ailments such as runner's knee or jumper's knee by strengthening the tendons around the kneecap.

This is due to the fact that balance training reduces the overuse or strain on those same muscles in exercises that rely on repetitive motions (such as jogging).

Improving these areas makes them not only stronger, but also more resilient!

If you want to start with balance training, there are many simple exercises you can do at home, and many of them don't require any equipment.

Enhances Agility

Agility is improved by balance training. You can enhance your agility by using a balance board or other equipment, which means you'll be able to improve your response time and coordination while simultaneously exercising the same muscles that help you run longer!

These include strengthening core stability (which is required for all types of movements, whether at home or in sports) and training the stabiliser muscles around the ankles, which are used during athletic motions such as jumping and changing direction swiftly.

Balance exercise promotes agility by encouraging people to use their entire body instead of just individual sections, which improves coordination as well.

It also doesn't have to take long: several exercises only take approximately 20 minutes per session but are really beneficial.

An exercise ball is a frequent example because it trains various parts of the body at once and can be done while watching TV, sitting on the couch, or even on the way to/from work.

As a result, you'll have a stronger foundation for both everyday movements and athletic performance—and who doesn't want that?

If you want to start with balance training exercises, consider standing yoga postures, plank variations (side planks!), single-leg squats, stability ball push-ups, or lunges.

Enhances Long-Term Health Effects

Balance training improves long-term health by strengthening muscles that aid in everyday motions as well as athleticism. Improving strength and agility lowers your chance of injury while also improving coordination, response time, and speed!

What are the two most crucial aspects of our bodies for our capacity to balance?
Balance is provided by our inner organs (the vestibular system).
Because they are filled with fluid, the semicircular canals and the otolith organs, known as the utricle and saccule, are important for our feeling of balance.
The fluid inside these canals moves when we move.
This movement then stimulates the balancing organs, which give signals to our brain regarding

where we're travelling in reference to gravity (up/down or left/right).

These balancing organs also operate with our vision; when you close your eyes while standing on one leg, it is more difficult to maintain balance than when they are open, because vision is important in balance.

If a person has poor motor skills or is unable to integrate all three types of vestibular sensory input—visual, proprioceptive, and tactile inputs—he will have more difficulty balancing himself and may be more vulnerable to falls that cause injury due to a weaker foundation.

How Can I Boost My Balance?

Walking, riding, and climbing stairs are all balance training activities that anyone may accomplish at any time and from any location. Yoga, balancing board exercises, and stability ball routines are all fantastic ways to improve balance and strength in the comfort of your own home without having to go to the gym! Stretching helps loosen tight muscles - Stretching before balance training helps loosen tight muscles that might create balance issues. Tai chi motions - Tai chi is a form of balance exercise that can be done in the comfort of your own home and at any time.

Balance board workouts - Include an exercise ball, balance board, or other device in your balance training for increased strength and injury prevention!

What would balancing training entail?
Exercises that promote balance are included in balance training. Because balance is a combination of strength, coordination, and agility, any workout that improves one or all of these will also help with balance!
Yoga postures such as tree pose (Vrksasana), in which you must balance on one leg while keeping the other extended out behind for an entire minute, help strengthen muscles in the

lower body responsible for balance and increase core stability because your centre must be strong enough to hold up against gravity when not using both legs at the same time.
In order to improve balance, there are different instruments available such as wobble boards/boards, balancing cushions/cubes, Bosu balls (a half ball with a flat bottom that may be stood on), balance discs, and balance plates.

What exactly is a coordinating system?
Our ability to integrate sensory information and use it to govern movement is described by the coordination system.

When executing balance exercises like walking heel-to-toe across a line, we rely on visual input from what's directly in front of us, proprioceptive (our awareness of where body parts are placed), and tactile (touch) inputs from skin receptors all at once.
If an individual lacks one sort of sensory input—visual, proprioceptive, and/or tactile—due to weak motor skills, he may find it more difficult to execute activities requiring coordination, such as walking heel-to-toe across a line.

What kinds of coordination exercises are there?

5 Coordination Exercises for Your Programming

Ball or balloon toss - Because you can only see the ball through your peripheral vision, this coordination exercise is excellent for building hand-eye coordination. This coordination workout can be done with one or two people who stand about seven feet apart and toss the ball back and forth using only their wrists (no arms).

Wrist to Wrist Pass - In this coordination exercise, you pass a volleyball or other object from one side of your body to the other using only your wrists (no arms).

Walking with Weights - Similar to walking while balancing on an unstable surface, this coordination workout combines upper and lower body strength to improve overall coordination!

Jump Rope - Jumping rope is coordination training that also helps with agility and endurance!

Juggling and dribbling a basketball, soccer ball or another object that needs coordination are also excellent techniques to improve coordination!

Balance training has been shown in studies to increase response time, strength, agility, and long-term health impacts.

With so many advantages to be gained from a simple activity like balance training, it's no surprise that it's a hot topic in the fitness business right now.

Balance training has been proved to improve concentration, which will assist you in avoiding injury by slowing down or pausing when necessary before putting too much weight on specific muscles or joints!

Remember, it doesn't matter how old you are; just start today to make tomorrow better!

I hope this has given you some useful information about the benefits of balancing training and how it can be an important element of your overall fitness programme.
By including balance exercises into your daily routine, you'll gain the benefits of a healthier lifestyle, such as greater energy levels and improved emotions!

•Easy balance exercises suitable for beginners.
Certainly! Here are some examples of beginner balance exercises:

1. Single-Legged Stand:

• Stand on one leg and lift the other slightly off the ground; if necessary, grab a chair or a countertop for support.

2. Walk from heel to toe:
• When walking in a straight line, place the heel of one foot directly in front of the toes of the other.
• Concentrate on keeping a straight course and a steady balance.

3. Toe tapping:
• Stand with your feet hip-width apart and softly tap one foot to the side before returning it to the centre.

• Repeat on the opposite side, alternating taps.
Swinging your legs:
• Grab a firm surface and swing one leg forth
and backward, keeping motions controlled and
progressively increasing the range of motion.

5. Tree Position:
• Transfer your weight to one leg, bringing the
sole of the opposing foot to the inner thigh or
calf (avoid the knee).
• Locate a focus point to aid in balance, and put
your hands together in front of your chest.

6. Leg lifts on the side:
• For added support, stand next to a counter or a wall.
• Lift one leg straight out to the side, then drop it back down.
• Repeat on the opposite side.

7. Marching in Time:
• While standing, lift your legs towards your chest.
• Maintain good posture and a consistent pace.

Remember to begin with activities that are appropriate for your present level of comfort and progressively progress as your balance improves. Always prioritise safety and feel free to seek assistance when necessary.

Chapter 6

Flexibility and Stretching

Flexibility is the ability of a joint or group of joints to move through an unrestricted, and preferably pain-free, range of motion, which is essential for good sports performance. Stretching and flexibility exercises maintain muscular function and enhance range of motion. Furthermore, training your body to be more flexible has numerous potential benefits, including lower chance of injury, enhanced strength, better posture, and improved balance.

Static stretching, dynamic stretching, active isolated stretching, and myofascial release are the four types of flexibility training. These flexibility exercises can be done alone or at the end of your existing workout sessions. Consistent stretching, like other training routines, will yield the best benefits and improve the rest of your fitness endeavours.

We will discuss how to become more flexible as well as how to incorporate stretching into your fitness routine. You'll find everything you need to improve your range of motion, eliminate stiffness, or simply improve your flexibility right here.

•Exploring the benefits of flexibility.

Flexibility is described as the ability of your joints and limbs to move through their whole range of motion. Because flexibility declines with age, it is critical to include flexibility activities in your training routine.

The Advantages of Flexibility

Flexibility is an essential component of good health. Tight muscles can create issues throughout your body. As you age, your muscles lose strength and size, and you become stiffer and less nimble. Stretching at least two to three times per week will help you gain flexibility.

There are numerous physical advantages to becoming more flexible and agile.

Protects against injuries

You will be able to handle more physical stress if you have developed strength and flexibility. If you are less flexible, you will be more prone to tendons, muscles, and ligament injuries. Failure to stretch and keep your muscles supple will cause the tendons around your muscles to harden. This reduces your range of motion, making it easy to go beyond what you can comfortably perform. This could result in strains, sprains, or even ruptures. Because of the increased range of motion, increased flexibility reduces the chance of damaging your muscles, ligaments, and tendons.

Less discomfort

Flexibility exercises will help to lengthen and open your muscles. This alone will make you feel better. Because your muscles are looser and more relaxed, you will have less pains and aches. This will

also result in less muscle spasms in your body.
Back discomfort can occur as a result of tight muscles in the back and lower body. Improving your flexibility will aid in the treatment and prevention of pain. Tight hamstrings can cause back pain by pulling the pelvis down, putting pressure on the lower back.

If you have trouble twisting your upper body from side to side, it is time to stretch your lower body muscles.
Improved posture and balance result from increased range of motion.

Increasing the flexibility of your muscles will almost certainly improve your posture. It will also enable you to be correctly aligned and fix any imbalances you may have. A greater range of motion will make it easier to sit and stand in certain positions.

Flexibility provides more than just better posture and a wider range of motion. It can make simple actions like reaching over to grab something or bending to choose something easier. It will also make exercise more convenient.

increased power

It is critical to improve your strength as you grow more flexible. To be strong and sturdy enough to support your body and its actions, your muscles should be able to withstand a respectable amount of tension. This allows you to be physically fitter.

improved physical performance

Physical performance will improve as your flexibility improves and your range of motion expands. Because of the flexibility exercise, your muscles will operate more efficiently.

Flexibility training is an important aspect of any workout regimen, as well as daily living. It has numerous advantages that will simply make conducting regular duties more comfortable.

•Gentle stretching routines to improve flexibility.

You probably stretch a little at the gym, but stretching is more than a pre-workout and post-run ritual. A daily stretching routine can improve your overall health by increasing flexibility, releasing muscle tension, and decreasing stress.

Are you ready to incorporate some daily stretches into your routine? Let's get started!

Stretches to do on a daily basis
- Head swivel
- Shoulder roll
- Triceps stretch
- Arms and abdominal stretch
- Standing quad stretch
- Standing hamstring and calf stretch
- Figure four
- Hamstring stretch
- Kneeling hip flexor stretch
- Child's Pose

The Advantages of Daily Stretching

Stretching not only feels great, but it's also excellent for you! Fitting a 10- to 15-minute stretch session into your daily routine has numerous health advantages.

Stretching can be used to:

Relax tense muscles. Are you stiff from your day job or workout? Stretching is an excellent approach to ease muscle stress and tightness.

Increase your range of motion and flexibility. Stretching improves the flexibility of your muscles and joints. Stretching can also improve your range of motion, according to a 2012 study. This can help you get bendy for yoga or simply move more effortlessly across your living room.

Improve your posture. Is bad workstation posture ruining your mood? According to a tiny 2014 study, stretching may help you be more conscious of your posture and minimise that forward sag in your shoulders.

Pain should be reduced. Stretching may help lessen pain caused by chronic diseases or injuries because it relieves muscle tension. Stretching, according to a small 2015 research, can also help alleviate discomfort while correcting poor posture.

Reduce your chance of harm. Working out or engaging in physical activity without a sufficient warmup can put you at risk of injury. A regular stretch session may aid in the prevention of strains and sprains.

Improve your circulation. According to a tiny 2013 study, stretching is an excellent approach to improve circulation. Better blood flow can also improve your general heart health, muscular recovery, and soreness.

Reduce stress. Stretching can assist reduce tension, resulting in a stress-free body and mind.

Relieve headaches. Stretching can help relieve headache-causing stress and bring sweet relief.

Your daily stretching routine of 15 minutes

You can perform stretching exercises whenever you want. However, two excellent times to incorporate movement into your routine are when you first wake up and before you go to bed.

A proper warmup is essential if you want to stretch around your training regimen — yet stretching alone may not be enough. However, studies show that doing dynamic stretches (active motions that create a stretch) before a workout and static stretches (holding one position for a long) afterward is preferable.

Try this combination of static and dynamic stretches to maintain your muscles slim and limber.

1. Head swivel
   - Stand tall, arms at your sides, and feet shoulder-width apart.
   - Lower your chin to your chest gently.
   - Complete a full rotation by slowly rolling your head to one side.
   - When your head is back at your chest, relax for 5 seconds before rolling to the opposite side.
   - Repeat 5 times more.

2. Shoulder swivel
- Stand tall with your arms at your sides.

- Raise your shoulder blades as if shrugging your shoulders, making sure to leave some space between your shoulders and ears.
- Shifting your shoulder blades back and forth
- Repeat 5 times in one direction, then 5 times in the other.

3. Triceps extension

- Place your feet shoulder-width apart and stand tall.
- Extend your right arm in front of you, then cross it in front of your torso.
- Bend your left arm and softly move your right forearm closer to your chest.
- Hold for 10-30 seconds before releasing.
- Rep on the opposite side.

4. Arm and abdominal stretches
- Place your feet hip-width apart and cross your right foot over your left foot.
- Raise your arms upward and grip your left wrist with your right hand.
- Lower your shoulders and lean to the right, leaving space between your ears. This stretch should be felt in your sides and shoulders without causing discomfort or tingling.
- Hold the position for 15 to 30 seconds.

- Return to a standing position and do the opposite side.

5. Quad stretch while standing
    - Place your feet shoulder-width apart and stand tall.
    - Raise your left foot towards your buttocks and hold your foot or ankle with your left hand.
    - Hold for 30 seconds before lowering your foot.
    - Rep on the opposite side.

6. Hamstring and calf stretch while standing

- Stand tall and place your right foot in front of your left foot.
- Flex your right foot while keeping your left heel firmly planted on the floor.
- Lean forward and grip your right toes with your left hand (for support, position your right hand behind your back).
- Take a 30-second break here.
- Return to a standing position slowly.
- Repeat on the opposite side.

7. Stretch figure four
- Lie faceup on the floor and lift your legs off the ground, bending your knees at a 90-degree angle.
- Place your right ankle over your left knee, then your hands on your left leg (just below your knee).
- Bring your leg closer to you until you feel a stretch.
- Hold for 30 seconds before releasing.
- Repeat on the opposite side.

8. Stretch your hamstrings.
- With your legs out in front of you, lie on your back. Bend your right leg in so that your foot rests adjacent to your left thigh.
- Position your hands behind your right thigh. Straighten your right leg, heel contracted, and bring it towards your body (stop when you feel a stretch in the back of your leg).
- Maintain for 30 seconds.
- Change legs and repeat. If it's difficult to reach your leg, try using a stretch strap or a towel.

9. Hip flexor stretch while kneeling
   - Kneel on the floor and step forward with your right foot, forming a 90-degree angle at your hip and knee.
   - Tilt your pelvis upward by using your core and glutes. A gentle stretch will also be felt in your left hip.
   - Maintain for up to 30 seconds.
   - Change legs and repeat.

10. Child Pose

- Begin on all fours on a mat, knees exactly beneath hips and toes pointing behind you.
- Sit back slowly, allowing your butt to descend towards your heels.
- Lower your chest to the floor, allowing your hands to slip forward.
- Maintain for 30 seconds to 1 minute.
- Relax for 10 seconds after releasing the stance.
- Repeat at least three times.

Stretching on a daily basis is an excellent approach to keep your body and mind in peak condition. You'll also benefit from enhanced flexibility, improved circulation, and stress relaxation (wow!).

We understand that including even a short stretching exercise into your day can be difficult. If you're seeking for solutions to stay on track with your #goals, consider the following:

Schedule your daily stretch session at the same time.

Begin with a 5-minute exercise and gradually increase to 10, 15, or even 30 minutes!

Change up the types of stretches to keep things interesting.

Stop stretching immediately if you feel any pain. Stretches should be pleasant, if not slightly uncomfortable if your muscles are tight, but they should not be painful.

Pay close attention to any sensitive areas and consult a healthcare expert if you suspect something is wrong or if you feel more "ouch" than "ahhhh."

Chapter 7

Cardiovascular Conditioning

•Introduction to cardiovascular exercises.

Your heart rate has increased. You exhale more quickly and profoundly. You also perspire. That's probably because you've been working the major muscles in your legs, arms, and hips for a long time. When these primary muscles are engaged in activity, the rate of breathing increases to produce energy. As a result of the increased need for oxygen, respiration and heart rate increase. This type of action is known as cardiovascular exercise, or cardio for short.

What exactly is aerobic exercise?

Cardiovascular exercise, often known as aerobic or endurance exercise, is any type of activity that involves aerobic metabolism. That is, oxygen is strongly engaged in the cellular activities that provide the energy required to sustain the activity during the activity. Your heart rate increases, and you breathe more deeply in order to maximise the amount of oxygen in your blood and help you use oxygen more efficiently. As a result, you are more energised and do not tyre easily.

Cardiovascular exercise is any strenuous activity that boosts heart rate and breathing while increasing oxygen and blood flow throughout the body by utilising big muscle groups repetitively and rhythmically. This type of activity gradually stresses your most essential internal organs and enhances the operation and performance of your heart, lungs, and circulatory system. Cardiovascular exercise benefits several facets of health, including heart health, mental health, mood, sleep, weight regulation, and metabolism.

With each beat, the heart becomes more efficient in pumping oxygen-carrying blood, the lungs become more efficient in taking in oxygen, and the muscles become more suited to use more oxygen. However, as your breathing and heart rate increase, the surge should not be so strong that you feel the need to stop and relax. If you have a strong want to stop and rest, unexpected pain, or alarming symptoms when doing cardio, such as fast walking, cycling, swimming, running, or speed climbing, you must stop immediately and seek medical attention.

To be termed cardio, an exercise must raise your heart rate and breathing rate to a moderate to strong intensity level (at least 50% of your regular rate) for at least 10 minutes. As a result, activities to develop strength, such as resistance exercise, utilising weight machines, lifting weights, and core workouts, are not classified cardio because they do not boost the heart rate throughout the exercise session.

What are the most popular cardiovascular exercises?

- Running
- Jogging or jogging in place
- Brisk walking Bear crawls
- Burpees
- Swimming

- Water aerobics
- Cycling and bicycling
- Dancing
- Cross-country skiing
- Racewalking Basketball, volleyball, soccer or racquetball
- Kayaking, paddling, or canoeing
- Rowing
- Circuit training
- Rope jumping
- Stair climbing, in-line skating, martial arts, golfing, hiking
- HIIT (High Intensity Interval Training), mountain climbing, jumping jacks, squat jumps, split jumps, roller blading, and

kickboxing are all activities that can be done on a regular basis.

The following equipment are the most commonly utilised for aerobic exercises:

- Treadmill
- Machine for stepping
- Cycles that are stationary
- Ski instructor
- Machine for rowing
- Elliptical machine
- Bike that reclines
- Bike that stands upright
- Staircase climber

- Ergometer for the upper body
- Wave-trainer
- Versa-climber
- AMT Precor

What are the many types of cardiovascular exercise?

Cardiovascular exercise is broadly categorised into three types: high-impact cardio, low-impact cardio, and no-impact cardio.

High-intensity cardio

High-impact cardio refers to any cardiovascular activity that requires you to lift both of your feet off the ground at some point during the activity.

It is also known as a weight-bearing exercise since you are using your limbs to maintain your own body weight against the force of gravity. Jumping rope, high-impact aerobic dance, and specific types of advanced strength training are all examples.

Low-impact cardio

Any cardiovascular activity in which one foot is always on the ground. However, low-impact cardio should not be mistaken with low-intensity cardio because many low-impact activities are intense. Low-impact cardio is still a weight-bearing activity that is beneficial for bone health as well as lung and heart training.

Walking, hiking, and low-impact aerobic dance are all examples of low-impact cardio.

Cardio without impact

Because being immersed in water diminishes the pull of gravity on the body, cardiovascular exercise performed in water is characterised as no-impact. Swimming and water aerobics are hence low-impact cardio workouts. Bicycling is also a low-impact cardio exercise because the bike's tyres and frame support the majority of the body weight. Cycling and swimming exercise are good if you have an arthritic disease or are recovering from an injury since they minimise most of the jarring and pounding associated with land-based cardiac activity.

What are the benefits of cardiovascular exercise? Cardio exercise involves moving the big muscles of your body for an extended length of time while keeping your heart rate at or near 50% of its maximal level. Regular aerobic exercise will strengthen your cardiovascular system, resulting in more capillaries supplying more oxygen to the cells in your muscles. You will also notice a gain in stamina and endurance with each session.

Cardio exercise has the following specific advantages:

Heart health has improved.
You can build stronger muscles, including those of the heart, that control your blood pressure, improve HDL (good cholesterol), reduce anxiety and stress, decrease blood proteins and fats that contribute to blood clots, prevent heart disease, and manage diabetes by engaging in 30-60 minutes of cardiovascular exercise daily.

Improved brain health
Regular aerobic exercise increases the volume or size of the brain areas that affect memory and

reasoning skills. Frequent cardiovascular activity also slows the pace of brain shrinkage in the elderly, boosting cognitive performance. However, cardio can also help you get a good night's sleep, which is essential for your mental health.

accelerated metabolic rate

All types of cardio boost metabolism by increasing the synthesis of Fibroblast Growth Factor 21 (FGF21) hormone, which boosts metabolism, suppresses appetite, and burns more calories.

Weight control

Cardio helps to burn excess calories and control weight by boosting the heart rate into the target heart rate zone, which is the zone where the body burns the most calories. Walking, swimming, running, and jogging burn a lot of calories over time, whereas moderate to high intensity cardio burns a lot of calories per workout session. Jumping rope, running stairs, walking, rowing, cycling, and high intensity interval training (HIIT) are all great cardio workouts for losing weight.

Enhanced mood and energy

Cardiovascular activity increases the secretion of endorphins, which are neurochemicals that generate euphoria. Cardio also increases the production of mood-enhancing chemicals like dopamine, serotonin, and norepinephrine. You feel more energised and ready to finish your normal activities when your mood improves. However, increased hormone release reduces stress, improves stamina, energy, and memory and mental focus.

Improved immune system

Regular exercise boosts the production of antibodies and white blood cells, which improves the body's ability to fight illnesses. The release of FGF21 also increases metabolism and strengthens the immune system. Cardio exercise actually protects the body from a variety of ailments, including hypertension, stroke, osteoporosis, diabetes, and heart disease.

Arthritis management

Through movement, cardiovascular exercise helps to alleviate the pain associated with arthritis and to reduce stiffness at the joint.

How should you perform cardiovascular exercise in order to get the most out of it?

For greatest advantage, you should engage in cardiac activity at least three times each week.

For example, if you have more time on weekends, you can plan the first two days to be Saturday and Sunday, then look for another day in the middle of the week. So you don't have to do all of your exercises on weekdays—though if you can fit them into your schedule, go for it. Cardiovascular exercise does not require long periods of time. Short bouts of cardio (as little as 5 minutes apiece) are just as effective as lengthier sessions, as long as the effort level and overall cumulative training time are equivalent. Twelve 5-minute spurts of high-intensity aerobics, for example, are as beneficial as a single 60-minute workout. If you're worried about your busy schedule, cardio is a terrific solution. A lot of cardio workouts also don't require any particular equipment or a gym membership.

For a beginning, low-to-moderate intensity sports such as walking, bicycling, swimming, dancing, running, martial arts, in-line skating, canoeing, golfing, and water aerobics are recommended. This will allow you to do things for longer periods of time and get additional health benefits. However, while selecting your hobbies, choose those that you enjoy so that you can stick to them as you go.

Furthermore, increasing the intensity of an activity over time is preferable to increasing the volume or length of the activity. Cardio should not be overdone, and spending hour after hour at a slow-to-moderate pace will not provide you with any additional benefits. So, after you can complete 30-45 minutes of an exercise 3-4 times per week, you should take it a step further and pursue its advanced principles.

The following are the fundamental guidelines for successful cardiovascular exercise:

Begin slowly.
Begin with the basics. Begin with a 5-minute walk in the morning, followed by another 5-minute stroll in the evening. After that, gradually add a few minutes and gradually

increase the tempo. You'll be walking for 30 minutes every day in no time. As you begin, think about activities that interest you and that you will be able to pursue without cost or time restraints. Hiking, jogging, cycling, rowing, running, and elliptical exercise are all viable possibilities. Remember, it is any action that causes your respiration and heart rate to increase!

Prepare yourself
Take 5-10 minutes at the start of each session to progressively rev up your cardiovascular system and boost blood flow to your muscles. Warming up entails performing lower-intensity versions of

the cardio activity you expect to perform. For instance, if you plan to go for a quick walk, you can warm up by walking gently.

Conditioning

Moving at your own pace, prepare your body to be able to complete at least 30 minutes of cardio per day. In order for cardio to benefit you, you must first increase your aerobic capacity by increasing your heart rate, breathing depth, and muscular endurance to the point where you can comfortably accomplish at least 30 minutes of your chosen exercise.

Calm down

Take 5-10 minutes to cool down at the end of each session. Stretch your calf muscles, upper thighs (quadriceps), lower back, hamstrings, and chest to calm down. This post-workout stretch will allow your muscles, lungs, and heart rate to quickly return to normal.

Cardiovascular exercise has long been recognised as the foundation of every good fitness programme and the key to living a longer, happier life. Its benefits are also spectacular, including increased mood, better sleep, and a lower risk of heart disease, diabetes, stroke, and certain types of cancer, among others.

•Beginner-friendly cardio routines (e.g., jumping jacks, high knees).

At-home cardio workouts are a great approach to fulfil these exercise goals because they do not necessitate a costly gym membership or any expensive equipment! These activities can enhance your heart health, burn calories, and even improve your mental health, whether you're a novice or a seasoned fitness fanatic.

We'll walk you through 14 of the finest cardio workouts and exercises for each fitness level that you can do at home.

1) Lunge Jumps two persons lunge jumping
Lunge leaps are an intense variant of the standard lunge exercise that adds to your cardio workout programme. This activates many muscle groups at the same time, including your quadriceps, hamstrings, glutes, and calves, offering a full-body workout.

To do a lunge leap, follow these steps:
1. Begin by standing upright with your feet hip-width apart.
2. Take a step forward with your right foot, bending your right knee at a 90-degree angle and lowering your left knee to the ground.

3. Push off with both feet from the lunge stance and thrust yourself upwards explosively.
4. Switch your leg positions while in the air, moving your left foot forward and your right foot back.
5. Repeat, landing softly on the ground with your left foot in front and your right foot behind you.

2) Jacks of All Trades
Jumping jacks are a tried-and-true plyometric workout that can be done almost anyplace. Jumping jacks raise your heart rate while also engaging muscles in your legs, arms, and core, giving you a full-body exercise.

To do a leaping jack:

1. Stand up straight, legs together, and arms at your sides.

2. Jump into the air while bending your knees slightly.

3. As you jump, spread your legs shoulder-width apart and extend your arms over your head.

4. Land lightly and immediately reverse the motion by jumping back up to the starting position. Repeat.

3) Climbers of the Rocky Mountains

Mountain climbers are a great aerobic exercise that works your core, upper body, and lower body all while raising your heart rate. They can be used as a warm-up exercise before indulging in other activities, or they can be incorporated into circuit training or high-intensity interval training (HIIT).

Mountain climbers should:
1. Begin in a high plank stance, hands shoulder-width apart and feet hip-width apart.
2. Bring your right knee to your chest while keeping your left leg straight.
3. Switch legs quickly, bringing your left knee to your chest and extending your right leg.
4. Continue alternating legs, moving quickly as if ascending a mountain.

4) Prone Knees

High knees are a high-energy cardio exercise that targets your lower body while also giving a fantastic cardiovascular workout.

To do high knees, follow these steps:
1. Begin with your feet hip-width apart and your arms by your sides.
2. Bring your right knee up to your sternum.
3. Lower your knee quickly and repeat with the other knee.
4. Repeat, alternating your knees quickly.

5) Toe Tapping

Toe taps are a simple yet efficient cardio exercise that targets your lower body while increasing your heart rate. Toe taps are performed as follows:

1. Face a firm raised surface, such as a step or bench, with your feet together and your arms at your sides.

2. Lift your right foot and tap the ball of your foot quickly on the elevated surface.

3. Immediately lift your right foot off the ground and return it to its starting position.

4. Repeat with your left foot, tapping the ball of your foot on the elevated surface and returning to the starting position.

6) Squat Jumps

Squat jumps are a plyometric activity that combines the benefits of squats and explosive jumps, making it an effective cardiovascular exercise and an excellent supplement to an HIIT session. Squat leaps are performed as follows:

1. Stand with your feet shoulder-width apart, toes turned out slightly, and arms at your sides.

2. Lower yourself into a squat position by bending your knees and pressing your hips back as if sitting.

3. As you reach the bottom of the squat, firmly explode upward, extending your legs and launching yourself off the ground.

4. Swing your arms high while in the air for momentum and balance.

5. Return to the squat position softly, bending your knees to absorb the impact, and repeat.

7). Burpees

Burpees are a difficult, high-intensity workout that stimulates the entire body and include various motions such as a squat, plank, push-up, and leap. Burpees are performed as follows:

1. Begin in a squat position with your knees bent, your back straight, and your feet shoulder-width apart. 2. Place your hands on the floor between your feet.

3. Return to a plank posture, keeping your body in a straight line from shoulders to heels.
4. Do a pushup by bending your elbows and bringing your body towards the floor.
5. Return to plank and leap your legs forward to the starting squat posture.
6. Jump into the air with your hands above your head from the squat posture. 7. Land with your knees bent, return to the squat position, and repeat the exercise.

8). Box Jumps

Box jumps stimulate these lower body muscles as well as your cardiovascular system, making it a fantastic cardio exercise. Follow these instructions to accomplish box jumps:

1. Begin by standing with your feet shoulder-width apart, facing the box.

2. Lower yourself into a quarter squat while bending your knees.

3. Swing your arms back to gain momentum, then swing them forward as you push through your legs and jump up.

4. Tuck your knees into your chest and lightly fall on top of the box, focusing on resting on the balls of your feet.

5. Return to the starting position by stepping or jumping down, achieving a controlled landing with a modest bend in your knees.

9) Rope Jump

Jumping rope is a basic and effective aerobic workout that can be done almost anyplace with little equipment. Jumping rope's rhythmic and synchronised action can also help you enhance your coordination, timing, and agility.

To try jumping rope, do the following:
1. Begin in an open environment with enough overhead space to support the hanging rope.
2. Hold the grips of a jump rope in each hand, palms facing towards your body. Allow the rope to trail behind you and make contact with the ground.

3. Swing your wrists forward and jump up with both feet together as the rope passes beneath your feet.

4. To absorb impact, land softly on the balls of your feet with your knees slightly bent.

5. Immediately after landing, leap again, and repeat.

10) Static Jogging

Jogging in place is a simple and effective cardio activity that gets your heart rate up and mimics the motion of jogging or running without requiring a huge outside space or a treadmill. To practice jogging in place, do the following:

1. Begin by lifting your right foot off the ground and bringing your knee up towards your chest, then your left foot.
2. Swing your arms back and forth naturally, opposite the movement of your legs, to improve rhythm and coordination.
3. Maintain a steady pace that is comfortable for you while continuing this alternate motion.

11) Fast Skaters

Speed skaters are a high-intensity cardio activity that simulates the actions of a speed skater on the rink. Speed skaters and other lateral activities have been demonstrated to improve agility and stability.

Speed skaters should:

1. Start by remaining with your feet shoulder-width separated.

2. Perform a lateral leap to the right, moving your weight to your right leg.

3. Bend your right knee and extend your left leg diagonally behind your body as you land on your right leg.

4. Repeat on the opposite side, propelling yourself forward with your right leg and leaping laterally to the left, shifting your body weight onto your left leg and extending your right leg diagonally behind you.

5. Repeat this lateral leaping motion, swapping sides with each leap, as if you were a speed skater.

12). Plank Jacks

Plank jacks are a cardio exercise that combines the plank's core-strengthening advantages with the cardiovascular intensity of jumping jacks. Plank jacks are performed as follows:

1. Begin in a high plank position, hands directly beneath shoulders, and body in a straight line from head to heels.

2. Starting in a plank posture, hop both feet wide apart, akin to a jumping jack, while maintaining your arms and upper body immobile.

3. Quickly return to the starting plank position by jumping your feet back together.
4. Maintain a strong plank position while continuing the leaping motion, alternating between feet wide and feet together.

13) Lateral Moves

Lateral shuffles are a cardio exercise that involves quickly and deliberately shuffling sideways. This exercise primarily works the lower body muscles, particularly the inner and outer thighs.

To do lateral shuffles, follow these steps:

1. Begin in a low squat position, feet slightly wider than hip-width apart, knees bent.

2. Step to the side with your right foot and swiftly shuffle your left foot to the side, followed by your right foot, remaining in a low squat position.

3. Repeat, this time leading with the left foot and walking in the other direction. Continue lateral shuffling, rotating the lead foot with each shuffle.

14). Tuck Jumps

Tuck leaps are a plyometric explosive workout that combines a vertical jump with a tucked knee position in mid-air. Tuck jumps are performed as follows:

1. Start by remaining with your feet hip-width separated and your arms by your sides.
2. Bend your knees and jump explosively upward, propelling yourself with your arms.
3. When you reach the apex of your jump, tuck your knees in as tightly as you can.
4. Land softly, with your knees slightly bent and your leg muscles absorbing the force.
5. Spring back up into the air from the landing position and immediately begin the next tuck jump.

5 Methods for capitalizing on Your Home Exercises

Here are some useful tips and strategies to help you get the most out of your at-home workouts:

Have a Separate Workout Area

When working out at home, it's critical to build a physical barrier between your workout area and the rest of your living environment. This isolation can boost motivation and assist you in developing a consistent fitness programme free of distractions.

Check that you are properly fueling your vehicle.

Fueling for workouts and maintaining healthy diet are critical, especially for aerobic exercise. Consuming a well-balanced diet rich in carbohydrates, lipids, and protein, which contains the amino acids required to develop and repair muscle, is critical.

Adequate diet aids in injury prevention and post-workout recovery. Consult a healthcare practitioner or qualified dietitian for tailored advice based on your individual nutritional requirements, fitness objectives, and any underlying health issues.

Monitor Your Blood Glucose Levels

Using a continuous glucose monitor (CGM) to track blood glucose levels during home exercises allows you to monitor your blood glucose levels in real-time, providing you insights into how your body responds to exercise and the influence it has on your blood sugar.

Warm-up and cool-down periods

Warming up and cooling down prior to and after workouts are critical components of a safe and effective exercise regimen. Warming up your body for cardiac activity helps prepare it by gradually raising your body temperature and increasing blood flow to your muscles.

Similarly, following your workouts with a short jog or stretching allows your body to gradually and securely return to its resting state. Proper warming up and cooling down can also assist prevent injury.

Hydration, Hydration, Hydration!

Staying hydrated is essential for peak performance and safety during workouts. Adequate hydration increases physical performance, assists your body in compensating for sweat loss, and promotes healthy cognitive function during exercise.

The amount of fluid you should drink depends on your workout intensity, length, environmental circumstances, and personal demands. Listen to your body's thirst signals and get personalised hydration advice from a healthcare expert or sports nutritionist.

Chapter 8

Crafting Your Healthy Diet Plan

A balanced diet is critical in the pursuit of maximum health and well-being. Let's get into the nitty gritty of balanced nutrition, with an example of a healthy diet plan, suggestions for creating your own plan, and a basic formula for creating a well-balanced menu.

Balanced Nutrition's Foundations: A balanced diet includes a variety of foods that provide critical elements to support overall health. The following are the essential components:

• Fruits and vegetables: They are high in vitamins, minerals, and fibre and serve as the foundation of a healthy diet.
Proteins are necessary for muscle repair and growth. Lean meats, chicken, fish, beans, and tofu are all good sources.
• Whole Grains: High in fibre and provide lasting energy. Brown rice, quinoa, and whole wheat goods are examples.
• Dairy or Dairy Substitutes: A calcium and vitamin D source for bone health. Choose low-fat or fat-free alternatives.

• Healthy Fats: For heart health, include avocados, almonds, seeds, and olive oil.
• Hydration: Water is essential for several biological activities, including digestion and overall well-being.

Example of a day's menu
Let's build an example of a healthy diet plan based on the basic principles of healthy eating; using it as a basis, you may vary the items and receive a fresh menu each time:

Breakfast:

• Muesli with sliced strawberries and chia seeds.

• One glass of low-fat milk or a dairy-free substitute.

Lunch:

• Salad with grilled chicken or tofu, mixed greens, cherry tomatoes, cucumbers, and a vinaigrette dressing; quinoa or brown rice on the side.

Snack:

• A handful of almonds and an apple.

Dinner:

• Baked salmon or a plant-based protein substitute; steamed broccoli, carrots, and sweet potato.

Making a Healthy Eating Plan:
Set specific objectives: Define your health and dietary goals, whether they are weight loss, enhanced energy, or overall well-being.

Determine Your Daily calorie Requirements: Determine your daily calorie requirements based on criteria such as age, gender, exercise level, and goals.

Balance Macronutrients: Aim for a balanced macronutrient distribution of carbohydrates, proteins, and fats. Individual needs should be considered when adjusting the ratios.

Diversify Your Food Options: Include a wide range of foods to guarantee a full spectrum of nutrients. Change up your protein sources, your vegetables, and your whole grains.

Mindful Portions: To avoid overeating, keep portion proportions in mind. To assess portions, use instruments such as measuring cups or visual cues.

Basic Balanced Menu Formula:
• veggies and Fruits: Half of your plate should be filled with colourful veggies and fruits.
• Proteins: Reserve one-quarter of your plate for lean proteins such as fish, chicken, beans, or tofu.
• Whole Grains: Set aside a quarter of the remaining quarter for whole grains such brown rice, quinoa, or whole-grain pasta.
• Healthy Fats: Include small amounts of healthy fats from sources such as olive oil, avocados, and almonds.

Food Quantity Calculation:

For one meal, use the following general recommendations as a starting point:

• Vegetables and Fruits: 2 cups leafy greens or 1 cup chopped vegetables/fruits.
• Protein: 3-4 ounces lean protein.
Cooked Whole Grains: 1/2 to 1 cup cooked whole grains.
• Healthy Fat: 1-2 tablespoons olive oil or a small handful of almonds.
A balanced diet plan requires careful consideration of your nutritional needs and goals. You will not only nourish your body but also enjoy the journey to optimal health if you embrace a variety of nutrient-dense meals,

maintain portion control, and incorporate a diverse range of flavours. Remember that the key to unlocking energy and maintaining a lifelong commitment to well-being is balance.

•Introduction to a balanced and sustainable diet.

Let's delve a little deeper into the area of balanced and sustainable diets.

Why Is Your Diet Your Workout Wingman?: Consider your body to be a high-performance vehicle; the gasoline you use is important. A well-balanced diet does more than just keep you fuelled; it's the secret sauce that complements your workouts. The perfect vitamin combination boosts your energy levels, aids recovery, and guarantees you're ready to face anything comes your way.

Let's speak about the basic components of a balanced diet now. We are not enrolling you in a difficult nutrition class. It's about eating a variety of foods, such as vegetables, fruits, lean proteins, and whole grains. It's like a vibrant array of nutrients that your body desires.

For the Win on Sustainability: This isn't a crash diet or a quick remedy. It's all about forming long-lasting habits. Finding a way to eat that you can continue with in the long run is what sustainability entails. There are no drastic limits, only a balanced approach that feels good and fits your lifestyle.

Unleashing Mindful Eating: Have you ever sat down with a plate and it's suddenly empty, and you're not sure how it happened? This is where careful eating becomes possibly the most important factor. It's about being present with your meal - savouring each bite, enjoying the flavours, and knowing when you're full. It's a game changer in terms of developing a healthy relationship with food.

Small Steps, Big Impact: The best part is that you don't require a complete makeover. Small, realistic modifications in your eating habits might lead to big results. It's all about figuring out what works for you and incorporating it into your daily routine.

•Instructions on how to incorporate healthful foods into everyday meals.

Eating healthily can be challenging. Especially in the midst of daily life's rush and bustle. When you're pressed for time, you don't always make the ideal dietary choices and rarely take the time to enjoy your meals.

Even if your day is hectic, eating healthy and making wise food choices should be top priorities. Your health and well-being are critical. Making the appropriate food choices will keep you feeling well and encourage a healthy, long life.

13 Ways to Eat Healthily and Consciously Throughout the Day

1. Consume your greens. Make a salad with it or add it to your morning eggs. Include spinach, kale, cabbage, swiss chard and rocket. There are so many delicious greens to choose from.
2. Have a smoothie. When ordering smoothies, look for extra sugar in the ingredients. Also, try

to include some vegetables. Spinach, kale, steamed and frozen zucchini, and frozen cauliflower can all be included. The list goes on and on.

3. Snack frequently. Allowing yourself to become very hungry will cause you to overeat at your next meal. Keep healthful snacks on available, such as almonds, fruit, beef jerky, veggies, and hummus.

4. Learn how to cook your favourite vegetables. Find your favourite vegetables and begin experimenting with them. Roast them with olive oil and salt, steam them, sauté them, eat them raw — whatever works best for you.

5. Drink plenty of water. Drink a glass of water before each meal. Water ought to be polished off previously, during, and after work out. Always keep a container of water with you.
6. Avoid skipping meals. Skipping meals can lead to overeating and make it difficult for your body to maintain consistent insulin levels.
7. Avoid eating processed foods. If you can't, make sure you read nutrition labels. Some items labelled "healthy" do not necessarily fit the bill. Examine the labels to see what's really in your food. The fewer components used, the better.
8. Eat consciously and sparingly. Take your time with each bite and chew slowly. Take short rests

in between bites. If you eat too quickly, you may not realise you are full and may overeat.

9. Keep unhealthy food and temptations away from the house and your workstation. When people are hungry, they tend to choose the most handy snack. You'll be OK if you keep the unhealthy foods out and load up on healthier munchies.

10. Limit your intake of sugary drinks and sodas. You'll be shocked at how much sugar is added to your food once you start looking for it.

11. Prepare meals at home. You will almost certainly use far less butter, oil, and salt than restaurant cooks who strive for exquisite taste. You are also more inclined to consume less

calories. Restaurants typically serve significantly greater portions than you would at home.

12. Prepare your meals. Make getting a healthy lunch out of the fridge a simple and convenient job. You will have some delicious, healthy dishes at your disposal if you prepare and plan ahead of time. It may appear to be a daunting process at first, but once you get used to cooking in huge batches, you'll never want to go back.

13. Avoid being a distracted eater. When you eat or watch TV, you are bound to be distracted, which leads to overeating and a lack of enjoyment of your meal.

Changing your routine might be a time-consuming task. You can start with a couple from the list above and add more as you go. Do what works best for you; there is no such thing as a one-size-fits-all approach to healthy eating.

Chapter 9

Staying Motivated

Motivation is what drives us to take action, yet staying motivated isn't always easy. Learn how to get (and stay!) motivated, as well as what to do if you can't seem to get into gear.

Motivation can be both positive and negative. Motivation is what propels you towards a goal, what gets you out of bed in the morning, and what keeps you pushing through a task, determined to accomplish even when things get difficult. However, motivation can be positive or negative:

Positive motivation focuses on the positive outcomes that will occur if you take action. 'Finishing this task implies I'm only a step away from being qualified,' for example.
Negative motivations are preoccupied with the negative consequences of inaction. For instance, 'If I don't do this homework within the next several hours, I'll flunk my course.'
Both negative and positive incentives can be beneficial in certain situations. It is, however,

much easier to do something because you want to rather than because you want to prevent a specific outcome if you don't. Negative motivation can make you feel helpless and may even diminish your motivation if you don't have a constructive plan of action.

•Strategies for maintaining motivation on the fitness journey.

Starting a fitness journey necessitates commitment, consistency, and motivation. Maintaining motivation might be difficult at times. I've certainly fought with it throughout my fitness adventure. So, whether you're just getting started or have been on your fitness path for a while, here are some of the finest strategies that have helped me stay inspired.

1. Set Specific and Realistic Goals: Setting specific, attainable, and quantifiable goals is essential for remaining motivated. Set a broad goal and then divide it into smaller milestones. This will help you to recognise your accomplishments along the route. Having defined goals to strive for gives you a sense of direction and progress.

2. Determine your Why:
What is your personal motive for starting a fitness regimen? Is it to boost your confidence, your health, or your energy levels? Discovering

your "why" will act as a constant reminder of why you began and will keep you motivated during difficult times.

3. Create a Friendly Environment:

Encircle yourself with individuals who will uphold and empower you on your wellness process. Join fitness communities, find a workout buddy, attend group sessions, or hire a trainer. Having a support system can help you stay accountable and motivated when you need it the most.

4. Monitor Your Progress:

Track your progress using a fitness journal, app, or wearable gadget. Tracking allows you to see how far you've progressed and provides proof of your efforts. To stay motivated, celebrate milestones and reflect on your accomplishments.

5.Change Up Your Workouts:

Monotony can suffocate your motivation. Experiment with new exercises, try new training courses, or explore outdoor activities to spice up your fitness routine. Variety not only keeps things interesting, but it also pushes your body in new directions, preventing boredom and plateauing.

6.Indulge Yourself:

Make a reward system for reaching your fitness goals. After reaching a goal, reward yourself with something you enjoy, such as a massage, a new workout clothing, or a weekend getaway.

Rewards give you a sense of success and something to look forward to.

7. Imagine Success:

Visualisation is an extremely effective motivator. Visualise yourself achieving your exercise objectives and noticing beneficial improvements in your body and overall well-being. Immerse yourself in the sense of accomplishment and allow it to drive your motivation throughout difficult times.

8. Have Fun with the Process:

Discover activities and exercises that you truly enjoy. When you participate in physical activities that you enjoy, you are more likely to stay engaged and motivated. Experiment with several workouts until you find the ones that you enjoy and look forward to each time.

9. Establish a Routine:

Getting into a regular workout routine can be life-changing. Schedule your workouts on set days and times, and consider them as non-negotiable appointments. Making exercise a regular part of your schedule creates a habit that requires less willpower to maintain.

10. Exercise Self-Compassion

Remember that every fitness path has its ups and downs. It is critical to be gentle to yourself, especially during times of setback or low motivation. Accept the journey as a learning opportunity and try not to be too hard on yourself. Recognise and celebrate even minor wins along the road.

•Setting realistic goals and tracking progress.

Setting exercise goals and keeping track of your progress are both necessary for success on your fitness journey. However, people frequently make the error of setting unrealistic goals, which leads to disappointment and dissatisfaction. Setting reachable objectives that are realistic for your body and lifestyle is critical. This procedure will show you how to set realistic exercise goals and track your progress to achieve the greatest outcomes.

1. Begin with a Well-Defined Strategy

Before you make fitness objectives, you should know exactly what you want to accomplish. Make a plan for what you want to do and how you intend to do it. Define your ultimate objective and then set modest, attainable goals to assist you get there. This will allow you to track your progress over time and make modifications as needed. You can divide your goals into categories like strength, endurance, and flexibility, or you can concentrate on individual body parts like your arms, legs, or core.

2. Make Your Objective SMART.
Make your exercise goal SMART when you establish it. Specific, quantifiable, attainable, realistic, and time-bound objectives. A goal should be specific in order for you to know exactly what you will be accomplishing. Measurable, so you may choose how to quantify your progress. Achievable, so that the objective becomes more realistic and reachable. Realistic, in the sense that you create goals that are both tough and achievable. Finally, it should be

time-bound because this provides a specific endpoint and drives you to stay on track.

3. Move Slowly

It's critical to take things slowly once you've set your fitness goals. Don't jump into the deep end. You should avoid pushing yourself too hard in the early stages of accomplishing your goal. Making tiny and steady modifications to your routine will benefit you and keep you focused on your trip. Take tiny measures and form the habits required to achieve your goals. You just have to take it one step at a time, whether it's starting with walking or increasing your water intake.

4. Monitor Your Progress
Tracking your progress is one of the most crucial components of accomplishing your fitness objectives. Find a method that works for you, whether it's via apps or a regular notebook. Tracking your progress will show you how far you've gone and what you still need to work on. You can track your progress by tracking your weight, body measurements, BMI, or even how you feel after working out. Tracking your progress ensures that you keep motivated and on schedule to reach your objectives.

5. Rejoice in Your Victories

Finally, you should rejoice in your triumphs as you work towards your fitness goals. Celebrating your accomplishments is an excellent approach to keep yourself motivated and focused. It could be a cheat meal, a spa day, or purchasing a new training attire. Celebrating your tiny wins will make your trip feel more satisfying, keeping you inspired to stay on track.

Getting in shape is a process that takes concentration, patience, and determination. Setting objectives and evaluating progress while remaining realistic with yourself is required. We hope that these five pointers will assist you in setting realistic fitness goals and tracking your progress for the greatest outcomes. Remember that progress is progress, and every minor win counts as an important step towards reaching your fitness objectives. Don't give up now. Maintain your efforts; you're worth it.

Chapter 10

Lifestyle Integration

The 'Lifestyle-integrated Functional Exercise' (LiFE) programme successfully reduced the risk of falling in older persons by improving balance and strength while also boosting physical activity (PA). The disadvantages of LiFE, which is generally offered in an individual one-to-one format, are significant human resources and expenses, which impede large-scale implementation ability.

What precisely is a healthy lifestyle?

These five areas were chosen because previous research has demonstrated that they have a significant impact on the probability of early death. These healthy behaviours were defined and assessed as follows:

1. Healthy diet, computed and scored based on reported intake of healthy foods such as vegetables, fruits, nuts, whole grains, healthy fats, and omega-3 fatty acids, as well as unhealthy food varieties, for example, red and handled meats, sugar-improved drinks, trans fat, and sodium.

2. A healthy physical activity level was defined as at least 30 minutes of moderate to strenuous activity each day.

3. A healthy body weight is defined as a normal body mass index (BMI) of 18.5 to 24.9.
4. Smoking, well, there is no such thing as a healthy amount of smoking. "Healthy" in this context meant never having smoked.
5. Moderate alcohol consumption, defined as 5 to 15 grammes per day for women and 5 to 30 grammes per day for men. One drink typically includes 14 grammes of pure alcohol. This is equivalent to 12 ounces of ordinary beer, 5 ounces of wine, or 1.5 ounces of distilled spirits.

•Integrating exercise and healthy behaviours into one's everyday routine.

Prioritising our health and well-being can frequently take a back place in today's fast-paced society. Exercise, on the other hand, is essential for sustaining a healthy lifestyle and improving general well-being. By including exercise into your daily routine, you can reap numerous benefits such as improved cardiovascular health, greater energy levels, improved mood, and better sleep. We will look at basic strategies to help you develop healthy habits and integrate exercise into your everyday routine.

Recognising the Importance of Exercise
Regular exercise is not only important for physical fitness but also for mental and

emotional well-being. Physical activity causes the release of endorphins, or "feel-good" hormones, which contribute to an enhanced mood and lower stress levels. Exercise also helps to maintain a healthy weight, lowers the risk of chronic diseases, and improves overall cardiovascular health. Exercise has a consistently favourable impact on our well-being, according to research. You can reap the benefits of a healthier and happier life by investing time and effort in exercise. To supplement your workout, Good Indian offers a selection of apparel tailored to complement your fitness goals.

Taking Stock of Your Current Lifestyle and Fitness Level

Before beginning to incorporate exercise into your daily routine, you should evaluate your present lifestyle and fitness level. Consider your regular activities and discover areas where exercise might be easily incorporated. Consider walking or cycling to work, taking the stairs instead of the lift, or indulging in physical activities in your spare time. Understanding your present fitness level can also assist you in setting realistic objectives and tailoring your exercise plan accordingly. Good Indian offers fitness materials and tools to help you determine your fitness level, so you can start your workout adventure with confidence.

Setting Realistic Objectives

Setting realistic fitness objectives is critical for remaining motivated and consistent. It is critical to make your goals SMART: Specific, Measurable, Attainable, Relevant, and Time-bound. Instead of a broad objective like "get fit," try for something more precise, like "complete a 30-minute workout four times a week." Setting reasonable and detailed goals allows you to track your progress and enjoy your triumphs along the way. Good Indian activewear can provide you with motivation and confidence as you go towards your fitness goals.

Finding Exercise Activities That You Like
Finding training activities that you truly enjoy is essential for maintaining a long-term fitness habit. Investigate several types of exercise to find activities that match your interests and preferences. There are numerous activities accessible, such as jogging, swimming, dance, weight training, and yoga. Good Indian's activewear line is created to accommodate various exercise methods, ensuring that you feel comfortable and confident during your workouts.

Including Exercise in Your Daily Routine

Including exercise in your everyday routine does not have to be difficult or time-consuming. You can find inventive methods to incorporate physical activity into your busy schedule if you make fitness a priority. Consider getting up earlier in the morning to fit in a workout, taking active breaks throughout the day, or participating in fitness challenges or programmes that fit your lifestyle. Good Indian's activewear gives you the comfort and flexibility you need to shift from daily activities to workouts.

Overcoming Obstacles and Maintaining Consistency

We frequently face obstacles that can undermine our enthusiasm and consistency in sticking to a workout plan. Lack of time, motivation, or access to fitness facilities are all common roadblocks. To overcome these obstacles, it's critical to plan ahead of time, find an exercise companion for accountability and encouragement, and consider home training choices when access to facilities is limited. Good Indian's sportswear is designed to adapt to various locations and workout conditions, allowing you to overcome any barriers that may arise.

Progress Monitoring and Milestone Recognition

Tracking your progress is a great method to stay motivated and track your progress. To keep track of your exercise activities, duration, and milestones, consider using fitness apps, wearable devices, or keeping a workout journal. You can celebrate your development and keep inspired to strive further by documenting your accomplishments. Consider rewarding yourself with new Good Indian clothing when you hit fitness milestones, adding style and confidence to your fitness path.

Incorporating exercise into your daily routine is a significant step towards developing healthy habits and prioritising your health. You may easily integrate exercise into your daily life by understanding the value of exercise, reviewing your existing lifestyle, making reasonable objectives, and selecting activities you enjoy. Remember that developing healthy habits takes time and work, but the benefits of better bodily and mental well-being are priceless.

•Long-term success and maintaining a fit and balanced lifestyle.
Health and fitness are essential for living a long, active, and pleasurable life. It is properly

claimed that health is the most valuable asset that a person may keep. Teachers assign this topic to their pupils in order to improve their understanding of remaining healthy and fit, as well as to raise awareness among others. It also helps in youngsters developing a healthy lifestyle. Simply said, being healthy and fit entails taking proper care of one's body. We must remember that a healthy mind can only exist in a healthy body. Good mental and physical health allows one to maintain the necessary energy level to accomplish success in life. We must all work hard to acquire good health. Protecting your body from hazardous substances, engaging in regular exercise, eating properly, and getting enough sleep are all vital aspects of living a healthy lifestyle. Being fit permits us to do our tasks without becoming drowsy, restless, or exhausted. A healthy and fit person can enjoy life to the fullest without serious medical or physical difficulties and.

CONCLUSION

And here we are, at the end of our fitness adventure in "Quick Workout for Beginners at Ease." Congratulations on reaching the conclusion – you've covered warm-ups, cardio, strength training, balance exercises, flexibility, and even explored the world of a balanced and sustainable diet. It's been quite a journey, hasn't it?

Reflecting on Your Achievements:

Take a time to consider how far you've come. Maybe you conquered a new exercise, increased your endurance, or simply made exercise a consistent part of your routine. Every step, no matter how small, is a win.

The Journey Doesn't End:

But hey, the journey doesn't end here. Fitness is a lifelong adventure, and this book is just the beginning. Whether you continue with these routines, explore new workouts, or set new fitness goals, remember that each day is a chance to enhance your well-being.

Maintaining a Balanced Lifestyle:

As we wrap up, keep in mind that maintaining a balanced lifestyle is about more than just exercise. It's about holistic well-being — physical, mental, and emotional health. Listen to your body, prioritize self-care, and celebrate the joy that comes from taking care of yourself.

You've Got This:

So, as you close this book, carry the confidence and knowledge you've gained. You've equipped yourself with the tools for a healthier, happier lifestyle. Whether you're stepping into a new chapter or revisiting these pages, remember: you've got this.

Thank you for joining us on this journey. Here's to a life filled with vitality, joy, and the ongoing pursuit of well-being. Keep moving, keep smiling, and embrace the incredible journey of fitness!

REVIEW

Dear Readers,

Your feedback means the world to us! If you've had the chance to dive into "Quick Workout for Beginners at Ease," we would love to hear about your experience.

Your insights can help future readers decide if this book is the perfect fit for their fitness journey. Whether it's a few sentences or a detailed review, your thoughts matter.

Did the exercises resonate with you? How has it influenced your approach to fitness? Share your story and let us know how the book has impacted your well-being.

Your reviews are not just feedback; they are a source of motivation and inspiration for both us and fellow readers. So, take a moment to share your thoughts and help create a community of individuals on the path to a healthier, happier life.

Thank you for joining us on this adventure!
Warm regards, Manuel N. Rank

www.ingramcontent.com/pod-product-compliance
Lightning Source LLC
Chambersburg PA
CBHW070648250726

48662CB00001B/27